500
NURSING
TIPS &
TIMESAVERS

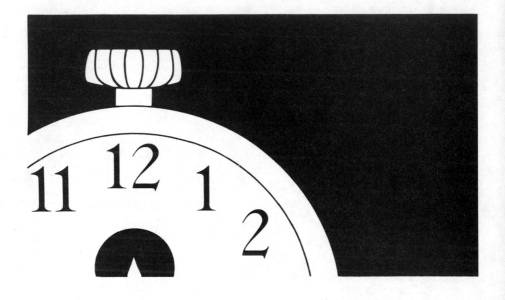

500

NURSING TIPS & TIMESAVERS

Quick and Easy Tips for Improving Patient Care

Nursing83 Books • Intermed Communications, Inc. • Springhouse, Pa. 19477

Nursing83 Books

Publisher
Warren Erhardt

Editorial Director
Eileen Cleary

Clinical Director
Patricia Nornhold, RN, MSN

Editorial Assistant
Garon Vogt

Designer
Edward W. Rosanio

Production Manager
Katherine Murphy

Art Production
Terry Gallagher, Craig Siman,
Joan Walsh

Proofreaders
David Beverage, Jane Doherty,
Gillian Gordon, Robin Miles

Typography Manager
David C. Kosten

Typography Assistants
Janice Haber, Ethel Halle, Betty
Mancini, Diane Paluba, Nancy Wirs

Intermed Communications, Inc.

Chairman
Eugene W. Jackson

President
Daniel L. Cheney

Production and Purchasing Director
Bacil Guiley

Copyright © 1982 by Intermed
Communications, Inc.
1111 Bethlehem Pike, Springhouse, Pa. 19477

ISBN 0-916730-52-2   TT2-7/83

CONTENTS

Quick Reference Guide

FOREWORD

It's time to give medications. Four call lights flash. And a patient codes. Who knows better than you how precious a nurse's time is?

To help you make the most of your valuable time, the editors of *Nursing83* have collected, reviewed, and organized the best *Tips and Timesavers* published in the pages of *Nursing* magazine. We've looked for better ways to help you do your work, to save you money, and to make every minute count.

The tips included in this book show how to organize equipment, administer medications, even keep your uniforms clean.

From the time you spend with patients to the time you spend keeping up with the changing profession, this book will help you save time. That's what the *Tips and Timesavers* are all about—saving time. And more time's something you can really use—isn't it?

The Editors

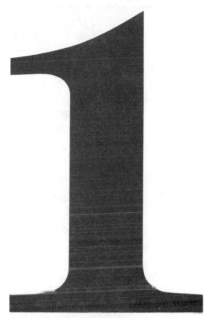

Don't discard—recycle

WELL-DRESSED FINGERS

Stockinette tube finger dressings can be used for more than just your patients' injured fingers. On *your* fingers, they're great for small swabbing jobs.

For instance, you can wear the dressings to cleanse your patient's outer ear or the folds around his eyes. You can use them to apply solvent to tape marks. And when necessary, you can wear the dressings over your gloves.

—ELEANOR QUIRK, RN

RESUSCITATED MANIKIN

When your resuscitation manikin wears out, here's how to replace the body. Remove its head and shoulders and disengage its chest mechanism. Then make a small slit inside the shoulder insert. Through this slit, tightly stuff Dacron batting (purchased at a local upholstery store) into the manikin's arms, legs, and abdominal area. After replacing the chest mechanism, continue stuffing until the manikin is filled. Put a vinyl patch over the slit in the shoulder to seal the stuffing securely.

Finally, reattach the manikin's head and neck band, and it is as good as new—but at a fraction of the cost of a new body.

—ANN P. MCCLELLAN, RN, BSN
GERRY TADLOCK, RN, BA

HANDY HOLDER

If you need a bedside dispenser for non-sterile cotton balls, try a plastic soft-margarine container. Cut a hole in the lid large enough to pull a cotton ball through. Then, fill the container with cotton balls and snap on the lid.

Besides being inexpensive, the dispenser's easy to use at a patient's bedside. Also, because it holds unused cotton balls in one place, it helps keep the patient's room neat.

—MariAnn Markan, BSN

WELL-DRESSED THIGH

If you have difficulty keeping a bulky dressing in place on a patient's thigh or groin, try using the panty section of a pair of panty hose.

First, cut off the legs and crotch. Then, slip the remaining panty section over the bulky dressing, with the elastic waistband toward the patient's foot. The panty section will hold the dressing in place without constricting circulation. It can be washed and reused several times before being discarded.

—J. Swenton, RN

PACKING IDEA

To pack deep, large wounds after irrigations or dressing changes, use a roll of sterile stretch gauze instead of 4x4s. Wearing gloves, hold the roll in one hand and a sterile hemostat in the other, releasing the dressing gradually and packing it in the wound. Since the stretch gauze is fluffier and smoother than 4x4s, it packs better. And because it's all one piece, the gauze can be removed easier and faster—a feature patients appreciate.

—Marie-Lise Shams, RN

FLOSS WORKS

When you need to secure a nasogastric tube but can't find any thread, use waxed dental floss. It's strong, and its convenient container keeps the floss clean while providing a handy cutting edge.

—Mary E. Anderson, RN, MS

INNOVATIVE IRRIGATING

If you don't have an eye irrigation tray, place a shampoo tray under the patient's head. The irrigating solution will run over the patient's eyes, into the tray, and off the edge of the tray into a basin or bucket at the bedside.

Your patient won't get soaked, so he'll be more comfortable, and you won't have wet towels or linens to change.

—Susan J. Birkholz, RN

TO A TEE

Surgical patients discharged with a long-term or permanent feeding tube, which must be clamped between feedings to prevent backflow, sometimes lose the clamp and are unable to find a replacement. A readily available substitute that fits perfectly into the end of a nasogastric tube is a plastic or wooden golf tee.

—D. Peters, RN

FROM SPOOL TO EXERCISER

Don't throw away those empty traction-cord spools. They make great grip exercisers for patients with spastic or flaccid paralysis of the hands.

Trim a spool's round cardboard ends to within ½ inch (1.3 cm) of the spool core, then cover the ends' raw edges with adhesive tape to protect them. Pad the core by winding cast padding or cotton batting around it several times. Secure the padding or batting with a layer of Elastikon, Coban, or other soft adhesive material.

Thread a long piece of gauze through the core's open center. Position the

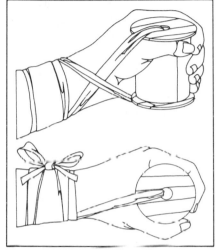

gauze so an equal amount extends from both sides of the core.

Now you're ready to attach the spool-become-exerciser to the patient's hand. First, pad your patient's wrist with a sponge dressing. Then put the core into his hand, cross the two gauze ends under his wrist, bring the ends up above his wrist, and tie them in a bow.

Depending on your patient's needs, you can use the exerciser one or more times daily.

—KATHRYN CALAMITA, RN

ON THE LEVEL

If long-term patients picnic on hospital grounds, finding level surfaces for their paper plates, cups, and utensils can be a problem.

To solve it obtain a large supply of empty fabric-bolt cores from a local yard goods store. Then cover the 30x18-inch (75x45-cm) cores with colorful adhesive-backed plastic paper. The result: lightweight, easy-to-clean, and easy-to-transport lapboards, usable by both wheelchair and ambulatory patients.

—ADA M. MASSA, RN

TRASH BAG TRANSFER

A large plastic trash bag will help you transfer a helpless patient from his bed to a stretcher. Just place the unfolded bag between the drawsheet and top sheet of the patient's bed, positioning it between the patient's shoulders and buttocks.

Because the plastic bag reduces friction between the sheets, you can grasp the drawsheet firmly and move the patient from his bed onto the stretcher with ease.

—DOROTHY J. LASALLE, RN

MULTIPURPOSE COVERS

Don't discard those plastic covers from 50-ml syringes. They can be used in many different ways at home or in the hospital.

Paint them brightly, for instance, and children will use them as crayon holders, sandbox castles, or bathtub submarines. Adults can use them to house crochet hooks or to organize sewing-basket spools. They're also great for storing sinkers, screws, and other tackle or toolbox items.

So next time, before you toss out the covers, consider their possibilities. How about using them to hold your toothbrushes when you go camping? Or to file all those coins you've been collecting. Or....

—PHYLLIS A. SMITH, RN

11

OVERBOARD

An ironing board makes a useful over-bed table for home-care patients. The board's adjustable, sturdy, and large enough to hold many of the patient's belongings.

—NANCY WESTERBUHR, RN, PHN

MORE THAN HEMS

A 6-inch (15-cm) hem gauge does more than just measure hems; it also helps measure the size of lacerations or contusions and the amount of bleeding or drainage on surgical dressings and casts.

Carry the gauge with you throughout the day—it takes up no more room in your pocket than a pen or bandage scissors.

—DIANE KLAIBER, RN

OINTMENT APPLICATOR

Add a disposable syringe (minus the needle) to your weapons for fighting decubitus ulcers.

Remove the syringe plunger, squeeze ointment into the syringe barrel, and replace the plunger. After cleaning the ulcer as ordered, squirt the ointment onto the ulcer. The pencil-thin ointment lines will allow you to target each crevice and fold.

—LYNDA L. SCHERFF, LPN

RED = CAUTION

While transferring a patient with a halo apparatus from his bed to a wheelchair, the metal rods on the apparatus may stab you in the head or chest.

To prevent this, cover each protruding rod end with a red rubber stopper from a blood-collection tube, then secure the stopper at its base with tape.

The bright red stoppers warn you to keep your distance from the rods, and if you still get too close, they cushion the blow. They also serve as conversation starters and tension relievers, encouraging patients and their visitors to smile and make the best of a difficult situation.

—MARGARET CAPITELLI, RN

ANY MESSAGES?

Looking for a fun way to encourage your depressed or unmotivated patients? Try "balloon" writing.

Inflate a nonsterile rubber examining glove and secure the opening with a knot or rubber band. Use a felt-tip pen to write a message on the glove, then tie or tape the glove to the patient's overhead bed frame, bulletin board, or other furniture. By combining wording such as "Happy Birthday," "Keep those feet moving," and "Cough, please" with diagrams, drawings, and smiling faces, you'll get your message across—even when you're not with the patient.

And when the patient's discharged, he can deflate his glove—*cum* balloon—and take it home with him.

—MARTHA G. OESTREICH, RN

NO MORE BATH BLUES

If a rheumatoid arthritis patient can't bathe himself, use a special bath sponge and heavy wire coat hanger. Stretch the top and bottom of the hanger. At the bottom, shape a triangle, stitch a folded sponge around it, and then fold a washcloth around the sponge. Adjust the hook at the top for the patient's best grip and bend the handle to suit his washing needs. If his elbows or wrists

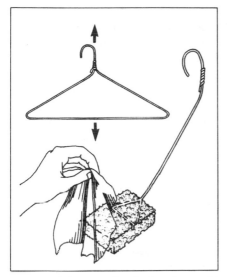

are too stiff to use the device, he could bend the handle into another position.

And how can a patient with stiff fingers squeeze out the sponge and cloth? Place the sponge against the side of the basin and press his hand flat against the sponge.

—LOUISE WIEDMER, RN

IN-THE-BAG SECURITY

If the plastic I.D. cards used for stamping charts, request forms, and hospital charges are insecurely clipped to patient charts, solve this problem by making a card holder from a used I.V. bag.

Cut off the label-pocket end of the bag, discarding the rest of the bag. Then, with a razor blade, cut through *one* thickness along the top of the label pocket, remove the I.V. label, and substitute it with the plastic card. Finally, tape the pocket to the front of the chart.

Tucked away in its pocket this way, the card is less likely to get lost.

—MARGARET E. SCOGGIN, RN

KEEP IT SIMPLE

Sometimes simple teaching tools are as effective as sophisticated ones. For instance, for a patient scheduled for a bowel resection, try this.

Take a flexible drinking straw and ask that he think of it as his large intestine. Tell the patient the flexible part represents the tumor that needs to be removed.

Then perform the "surgery." Cut the straw on either side of the "tumor," remove the tumor, and tape the straw back together again.

—JANE GRABENSTEIN, RN

IN LARGE MEASURE

Tape measures sometimes aren't long enough to measure large abdomens, so use twill tape instead. Wrap the twill tape around the patient's abdomen, mark the tape with a pen or pencil, then measure it against the patient's own tape measure. After determining the patient's girth, throw the twill tape away to prevent cross-contamination.

—MARIE FAIT, LPN

ON GUARD

Cover the ends of your hemostat with a *rubber* needle guard. The needle guard protects your pockets—without affecting the hemostat's clamping action.

—BETTY FRANCIS, LPN

HOORAY FOR THE FLAGS

With a little imagination, the "flags" on charts for stat orders can be used in many different ways. For instance, use them for evacuation drills. Put one—gray side out—on the outside door frame of the resident's room, then, during a drill, after making sure the room is empty, switch the stat flag to the red side.

—SR. SEAN DAMIEN, RN

COTS FOR CUTS

Want yet another use for rubber fingercots? They keep cuts on your fingers dry and clean as you bathe patients. The cots don't restrict your movement or offend the patient as rubber gloves might, and they cost less, too.

—MARY LU RANG, RN, BSN

SHOCK STOPPER

To protect patients with temporary pacemakers from electric shock, cover the pacemaker's unconnected wires with rubber tops from used Tubex syringes. The rubber tops ground the wires and can easily be removed when the wires are needed.

—BERNIE STREMIKIS, RN, BSN

SKIN SAVER

If diarrhea is irritating your patient's skin, suggest that he use a peri bottle (the kind given to new mothers for perineal care during the postpartum period). Tell him to clean his perineum with fluid from the bottle instead of wiping with tissues.

To use the bottle, he simply fills it with warm water (and some soap, if desired) and directs the water over the anus and perineum. Then he can blot the skin dry.

Caution: Tell the patient to store the bottle with the cap off, to discourage bacterial growth between uses.

—BARBARA J. SMITH, SN

MEALTIME AID

If a home-care patient has trouble taking fluids, use a meat baster to increase his intake.

Place the baster in the side of his mouth and squirt a small amount of fluid at a time. Hold a bowl under his chin to catch any spills. The baster accommodates pureed foods as well as fluids and is marked with ounces so you can note the patient's intake. Afterward, it's a handy tool for rinsing the patient's mouth, too.

—SANDRA CHIRO, LPN

A PEN POINTER

If you like to keep two different colored pens on hand together but need a penholder that protects your uniform from unsightly ink spots, try this:

Measure and cut some used I.V. tubing about 20 inches (50 cm) from the drip chamber. Then cut the drip chamber in half. Cover the points of two pens

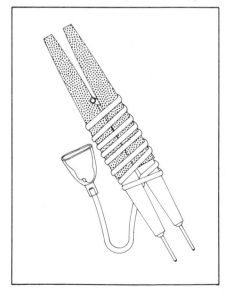

with the drip chamber and wrap the rest of the tubing between and around the pens to prevent unraveling (see illustration).

This penholder keeps your pens together and keeps the points covered. Best of all—no more ink-soiled uniforms to worry about.

—EVA TAPOLER, RN

A CALAMINE FIND

Instead of using a new cotton ball each time you apply calamine lotion for sunburn or minor skin irritation, try using—and reusing—an old roll-on deodorant bottle. Just clean and dry the empty bottle, fill it with calamine lotion, and roll the lotion onto the patient's affected skin. The rolling ball spreads the lotion evenly—without wasting cotton balls. After each application, snap off the bottle's ball for cleaning.

—JOANNE KRISKO, RN

IMPROVED WALKER

Help a patient with a walker become more independent and surefooted by buying a bicycle basket and attaching it to the front of his walker. He can then go to stores by himself and carry his packages home in the basket. And he'll become much steadier, thanks to the increased practice and exercise.

—SUZANNE DEVINE, RN

RECYCLED SOCKS

Worn-out tube socks can find new life as elbow protectors. Just cut off the leg portion and fold it in half to create a slip-on elbow guard.

These recycled socks contour to fit the patient's arm snugly, helping prevent skin irritation or possible ulceration from bed linens. Not only are they less expensive and more comfortable than disposable elbow protectors, they are also cooler, and easier to wash than sheepskin protectors.

—ELIZABETH A. FARMER, RN

MEASURE FOR MEASURE

Here's a way to help a homebound patient on fluid restrictions keep track of his daily intake. Mark a pitcher, bucket, or some other household container at the level showing his total daily allowance of fluids. Then tell him whenever he drinks some fluid, he should pour an identical amount of water into the marked container. This way, he can see at a glance how his intake compares to his total allowance.

—LINDSAY LAKE, BSN

"NET" WORK NEWS

With 4x4-inch (10x10-cm) stretch gauze bandages, use a short piece of 3-inch (7.5-cm) stockinette to wrap rubber ice collars.

With a pair of scissors, you also can turn stockinette into "mittens" for patients who try to pick at their dressings or drains.

—RACHEL PURNER, RN

TABLETOP VIEWS

At an extended care facility brighten patients' chair-tables with cheerful pictures of flowers, animals, and children. Cut the pictures from old magazines, arrange them on the chair-tables, and cover the tables with plastic wrap for waterproof protection.

Changing the pictures with the seasons not only perks up patients' morale, but also helps disoriented patients keep track of time.

—MARY E. REMMEL, LPN

NOW YOU SEE IT

To keep your Kardex from becoming a mess because of constantly changing orders, recycle unusable X-ray films into an eye-catching file.

Cut the clear films into 5x7-inch (12.5x17.5-cm) pieces and put them in the Kardex. Write orders from patient charts on the film, using a china marker. When orders are completed, just rub them off with a tissue or cotton ball.

With this system, new orders are more visible to nurses on all shifts.

—MARY ANNE FLOWERS, LPN

COVER STORY

The recorder and metronome switches on manikins for cardiopulmonary resuscitation instruction get a lot of use— and abuse. Not only do the knobs sometimes break off in the middle of a class, but they're very hard to replace.

Here's how to make your own replacement knob: Break off the needle of a disposable (preferably 25-gauge) needle at the hub. Trim the plastic hub at the syringe site, leaving the cover intact. Fit the cover over the broken switch, and you'll have a durable, inexpensive replacement knob.

—SUSAN SCHULMERICH, RN

CAST CARE

Here's a tip to pass on to patients wearing arm casts.

If the cast snags clothing and furniture, make a cast cover from an old nylon stocking. Cut the stocking's toe off and cut a hole in the heel. Then pull the stocking over the bulky plaster, poking the patient's thumb through the hole in the heel. Trim the stocking to about 1½ inches (3.8 cm) longer than the cast and tuck this end of the stocking under the cast's edge.

—CYRENA GILMAN, RN

DENTAL ASSISTANT

Here's a tip to pass on to postoperative dental patients. If bleeding occurs at home, and the patient has no gauze on hand, he can use a tampon instead. Tell him to just cut the tampon in half, place one half at the bleeding site and bite down. This will stanch the bleeding and save a phone call to the dentist.

—LYNNE COLE, RN

CARD GUARD

If your hospital's isolation cards identify only the type of isolation on the front and have specific isolation procedures listed on the back, to read the precautions on the reverse side, you must tear the card from the door—perhaps destroying the card.

Instead tape or hang on the door a 6x9-inch (15x22.5-cm) clear plastic pocket envelope (available in most stationery stores). The isolation card can be placed in the envelope but can be removed for reading without being destroyed.

—LOUISE M. LAND, RN, BS

HOMEMADE HANGER

Home-care patients who use wheelchairs or walkers to get around may also have catheter or urinary drainage bags.

Finding a place to hang the bags when the patients want to move around may be a problem. Use this idea:

With wire cutters, clip the bottom rung from a wire clothes hanger. Spread the two sides straight out and bend both

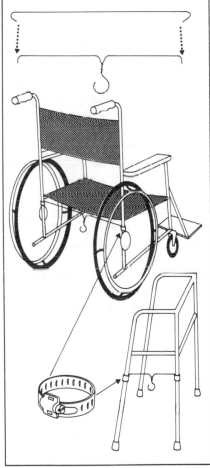

ends down 1½ inches (3.8 cm). Attach the wire, hook side down, to the walker or wheelchair with a pair of radiator clamps. Hang the catheter or drainage bag on the hook.

This wire hanger is sturdy and en-sures good drainage with no backflow.

—AGNES MOORE, RN, BSN

FINGER SPLINTERING GOOD

In an emergency, a hollow roller-type hair curler or the top half of the clamp-on curler will make a sturdy finger splint or protector for an injured finger.

—KATHLEEN CRUZIC

PAINLESS REMOVAL OF PAINT

To remove oil-base paint from the body, most people think first of using the sol-vent, turpentine. All well and good, but turpentine cannot be used around the eyes or mouth, for it can irritate and hurt. That doesn't help matters, espe-cially with children, who are apt to have wiped their eyes with paint-covered hands anyway.

To solve this problem, use mineral oil. It's nonirritating and effectively re-moves paint.

—PATRICIA L. BADOWSKI, RN

ONE SIZE FITS ALL

Custom fit disposable sponge slippers to a patient's foot size. Just tie a rubber band around the excess sponge at the slipper's heel, and it fits perfectly.

—PEGGY YOUNG, RN, BSN

SEAL 'N' SIP

Many patients who lack complete hand control and need to be fed, express the desire to feed themselves. Here's how they can drink from a cup without as-sistance.

Tupperware sells a "sipper seal," which is 85% spillproof. A set of two seals and four mouthpieces costs about a dollar. The seals fit over inexpensive Tupperware cups. Patients may drink right from the mouthpieces or through a plastic straw inserted in the mouthpiece.

—VICTORIA PAUL, LPN

EXPEDIENT EXTRACT

Liquids and tablets for deodorizing ostomy appliances are sometimes expensive and ineffective. Vanilla extract is an effective and inexpensive alternative. Instruct patients to saturate a small wad of tissue with vanilla extract and place it in the bottom of the appliance. They can repeat this procedure as often as necessary—every time they empty the appliance, if they desire.

—DIANE DEEGAN-MCCRANN, RN, ET

RIM WRAP

Patients confined to wheelchairs may complain about cracks and flakes in the chrome hand rims attached to the large wheels. To prevent this deterioration and the subsequent trauma to the hands, cover the rims with tubing. Cut a piece of clear, thick, polyethylene tubing lengthwise and slip it over the hand rim. Not only does it protect the chrome, but it also makes the rim easier to grasp and less cold to the touch.

—MELINDA CRAWFORD, RN

WORKABLE WALKWAY

Here's an economical way to help hip surgery patients, stroke patients, and others practice walking in their own homes. Arrange six or eight sturdy chairs, such as dining room chairs, side-by-side in two rows so their backs form a pathway. The patient can practice walking with the same support he would get from parallel bars.

—TERESA ROSE, RN

OUT OF THE CRIBS OF BABES

Crib blankets or coverlets are a perfect size for covering the laps and legs of people in wheelchairs. They're soft, washable, colorful—and they protect your patients' legs from cold and drafts.

—MARY HENDELA, RN

LOOK...NO HANDS

Teaching insulin injections to diabetics with blurred vision is always a problem. Since they need both hands to work with the insulin bottle and syringe, they can't hold a magnifying glass, too. Use a magnifying glass holder that's easy to make and inexpensive.

Stack five paper foam cups upside down, one on top of another. Punch a hole the size of the magnifying glass handle through the center of all five cups. Then insert the handle through the hole. Put the insulin and syringe in back of the magnifying glass. You can adjust the height by placing books under the cups.

A tall, narrow-necked bottle can also be used as a holder.

—LEE KORELITZ, RN

ONE-HANDED BANDAGE

Here's how to make a one-handed elastic bandage.

Sew a loop on one end of the bandage. Have the patient slip the loop over his foot as if he were putting on a sock, then wrap the remainder of the bandage around his leg. Not only does this decrease edema but also makes the patient more independent.

—JOYCE MEYERS, RN

MOUTHGUARD MAGIC

If a comatose patient with cerebral hemorrhage continually grinds his teeth and bites his lower lip, prevent further damage by using a football mouthguard. Soften it in warm water, and fit it over

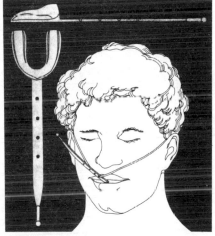

his lower teeth. Next, thread trach tape through the first hole of the guard's 6-inch (15-cm) helmet strap. Finally, run one tape end over each ear and tie the ends behind the patient's head—loosely enough to be comfortable, but tightly enough to hold the guard in place if he coughs.

You can buy the guard at most sporting goods stores.

—TINA SYKES, LPN

TUBE THERAPY

Don't throw away leftover pieces of Penrose drains; give them to the occupational therapy (OT) department.

In OT, patients with arthritis or those recovering from strokes can cut the pieces of tubing into various sizes. Such therapy not only exercises patients' hands but also provides the hospital with a supply of strong, flexible rubber bands.

—JOSEPH GLINSKY, ORT

HOSE POWER

Here's a way to recycle old panty hose. After laundering, slip one leg of the panty hose into the other and roll it up from waist to toe for storage. In an emergency, you can unroll the hose and use it as a pressure bandage for ruptured blood vessels, as a support wrap for sprained joints or torn ligaments, or as a sling for injured arms.

—SYLVIA MCINTYRE, RN

COMFY CRUTCHES

When a patient is discharged on crutches, give him a pair of disposable, stretch, foam hospital slippers. Not for his feet, though. Instead, fit the slippers snugly over the tops of his crutches to cushion his underarms and protect his clothes.

—IRENE STORMS, LPN, SN

AN I.D. TO RUN WITH

If your patient jogs, tell him to save his hospital identification bracelet when he's discharged. Usually, it'll list his name, address, phone number, allergies, and doctor's name. If not, he can ink in the missing information, then attach the bracelet to the ties on one of his jogging shoes.

This way, he'll always have identification with him, which could come in handy in an emergency.

—KATHLEEN E. MASON, RN

LIGHTWEIGHT CLAMP

Use umbilical cord clamps on nasogastric and "G" tubes. You'll find them lighter and easier to fasten and unfasten than the Hoffman and other heavy clamps.

—JO GOLDMAN, RN

PLAIN DRAIN

Used I.V. bottles are a boon for measuring gravity drainage from Levine tubes and the like. Be sure to wash the bottle first and remove the metal part of the cap. Leave the rubber stopper in the bottle and attach it to the patient's drainage tube.

The markings on the bottle will show you the amount of drainage, so you won't have to empty the bottle to measure it. To keep track of the amount over a period of time, mark the bottle with tape each time you measure.

If the patient's drainage tube is too short, you can use I.V. tubing to lengthen it. If drainage is too thick for I.V. tubing, use the regular drainage tube but attach it to a Foley catheter bag rather than an I.V. bottle.

—MRS. R. HAGER, LPN

NONSLIP SLIPPERS

Shiny hospital corridors can be hazardous to unsteady, recent postop or elderly patients. To help keep them from skidding—and boost their self-confidence—attach skid-proof bathtub appliqués to the soles of their slippers. Or you can put stockinettes on the patient's feet and attach the appliqués to the bottoms.

For pediatric patients, apply the appliqués to the bottoms of pajamas that cover the feet. To reinforce the appli-

qués so they'll withstand several washings, sew all around the edges.

And here's an even more economical tip—buy sheets of rubber that have an adhesive backing and cut out your own appliqués. Children love choosing their own designs—and they're a big boost to safety.

—ELLEN ROBEN, RN

ENDING EPISTAXIS

It's awkward enough for a nurse to apply pressure to a patient's bleeding nose, let alone having the patient do it himself.

From your inhalation therapy department, borrow a noseclip—the ones used during IPPB treatments and pul-

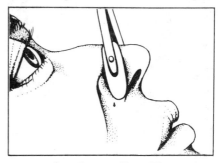

monary function studies. These exert the pressure needed to stop the bleeding.

—MARGARET A. POWERS, RN

SITTING COMFORTABLY

If you're caring for patients who've had rectal or perineal surgery, here's a way to help them to sit up straight and to increase sitting time without added pain.

Get a piece of foam rubber measuring about $14 \times 18 \times 4$ inches ($35 \times 45 \times 10$ cm). Cut out a circle in the center. Place the foam pad in a pillow case and let the patient carry it with him from place to place for his sitting comfort.

Patients claim this type of pad is more comfortable than pillows or rubber rings, and it's less expensive than many commercially made decubitus pads.

—MARIE RAY KNIGHT, RN

OUTPATIENT I.D.

An aphasic patient who has to come for speech therapy on an outpatient basis may want to keep his hospital I.D. bracelet and continue to wear it. If anything happens to him outside the hospital that he can't explain, he'll be brought to the hospital. And his name and hospital number on the bracelet will give the emergency department staff the needed information in a hurry.

—JACQUELINE BIRMINGHAM, RN
DONNA ARSEGO, SN

TEACHING TOOL FOR TRACH TECHNIQUES

Here's how to make an inexpensive yet realistic simulator for teaching tracheostomy care techniques.

Get an inexpensive Styrofoam head (the kind used to store wigs), and cut a hole an inch and a half in diameter at the site of the usual tracheostomy. Apply a thin layer of clear nail polish around the hole to prevent the Styrofoam from crumbling. If you're artistically inclined, you could paint a face on the head.

You can use this simulator to teach sterile dressing change technique, removal and cleansing of the inner cannula, sterile tie change technique, and inflation and deflation of the tracheostomy cuff. And, you can apply the various antiseptic agents used in tracheostomy care to clean the Styrofoam without causing it to deteriorate.

The simulator is so inexpensive and easy to store that you might want to get multiple heads to allow individual practice.

—ROSEMARIE MOORE, RN, BSN

EYE-OPENER

Need to improvise an eye cup if one isn't readily available? Use a sterile spoon—either teaspoon or tablespoon size. Fill the spoon with the eye wash solution. As the patient bends his head forward, place the spoon over the eye with the point resting on the inner corner of the eye. Then tell the patient to tip his head backward, open his eyelid, and wash the eye.

Your patient can use this improvisation at home or even away, as on a camping trip, for example.

—LADONNA KOLMAN, RN

AN IMPROVISED OVER-THE-BED TABLE

To make an improvised over-the-bed table, select a strong cardboard box large enough to hold a bed tray at a comfortable height for the patient. If the box is too tall, cut it down to size. Then cut out enough room for the patient's legs to fit comfortably underneath.

The box can then be used as is. Or it can be covered with a colorful self-adhesive paper for easy wipe after use. Young patients enjoy decorating this piece of "furniture."

—LINDA N. GUNBY, RN

21

FROM THE MOUTHS OF BABES

If your elderly or paraplegic patients have trouble retaining enemas because they lack muscle control, try cutting the tip off a baby bottle nipple and inserting the enema tube through the nipple.

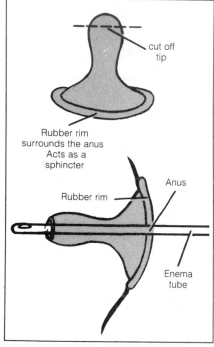

cut off tip

Rubber rim surrounds the anus Acts as a sphincter

Anus

Rubber rim

Enema tube

When the tube is inserted in the patient, the nipple rim surrounds the anus and acts as a sphincter.

—RAMONA CHISHOLM, RN

RESTRAINING PANTS

Patients may try to slip out of vest or belt restraints, and end up with the restraints around their necks or faces.

So, try a fashionable approach to the problem. Buy inexpensive cotton slacks and insert ties made of heavy twill tape (like venetian-blind tape) into the side seams at hip level. These ties replace the restraints, and keep patients in place effectively. What's more, they look better, too.

—SHARON MAYLOCK, RN

CUSTOMIZED CHAIR

If a patient constantly gets his arms and legs stuck in the side openings of a geriatric wheelchair, solve the problem by using plywood inserts to fit the chair sides. Make long, narrow pillows to pad the plywood. Then the patient has freedom of movement, and can't get himself into dangerous positions.

This idea can be adapted to other situations, too. For instance, make "bumper pads" from pillows to cover the side rails of the patient's bed.

—RUTH GAULT, RN

GRIPPING SOLUTION FOR ARTHRITIC HANDS

Many patients with arthritis in their hands have trouble gripping eating utensils, pens and pencils. To enlarge the grip on these and other slender items, use foam cylinders from hair curlers. A package of 10 or so costs about a dollar and they're available in many drug and department stores. Just slip the foam cylinder off the plastic curler spindle and onto the slender pen or handle.

—MRS. EVELYN ROSSKY, OT

HANDY SLIPPERS

Do you ever have trouble retrieving patients' slippers lying halfway under the bed? Try bending both corners of a wire coat hanger upward, then bend the hook one quarter of the way around.

Hang the slippers on the turned-up corners and hook the hanger to the bedframe. That way, the slippers are always handy.

—CATHERINE RAIDY, LPN

MATTRESS MANIPULATION

Here's a number of ways to recycle a Stryker foam mattress after a patient no longer needs it. First, send it to the laundry, where it is washed and dried. Then cut and use it in various ways.

Here are some:

—pads for wheelchairs (they take a lot of pressure off sore hips).

—wedges the size of a child's leg. Taped just above and below the knee, they serve as a restraint during clysis. They are soft and the child can still move his legs.

—pillows for positioning patients.

—strips that can be rolled to fit a patient's hand and used for exercising in physical therapy.

—JANE RAYBURN, RN

AN AID FOR PARTIAL SOAKING OF THE FOOT

Soaks are sometimes prescribed for the patient with a plantar wart on the ball of the foot. When using an irritating substance such as dilute formalin solution for soaking, you'll want to minimize damage by limiting the area of surrounding healthy tissue in contact with the solution.

So have the patient get a paint pan—the kind used when applying paint with a roller. Have him pour just enough solution into the deep end of the pan to cover the ball of the foot while the heel rests comfortably on the slanted

pan bottom, high and dry. The technique works just as well for soaking the heel while keeping the toes dry: just turn the pan around and put the heel in the deep end.

—BARBARA McVAN, RN

NEAT SHEET

Here's an alternative to rigid, wrinkled, uncomfortable plastic sheets that don't stay tucked in. Use a flannel-backed, rectangular vinyl tablecloth. To make it fit the bed properly, make some minor alterations.

First, cut about one third off the longest side of the cloth. Then cut this piece

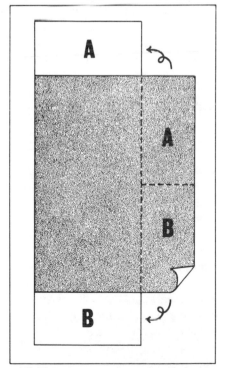

in half and sew one half to each end of the tablecloth. Attach these pieces so that the flannel side of the tablecloth and the vinyl sides of the two extensions are all facing the same direction.

Now the patient rests comfortably on the flannel side of the machine-washable, waterproof sheet, and the ends stay tucked under him *and* his bed.

—JESSIE BATEY
MAUREEN C. ORGAN, RN

FEEL THE WAY

If the beds on your unit are equipped with a panel of buttons for turning on the TV, calling the nurse, and so forth, vision-impaired patients may have trouble: turning on their TVs instead of calling you, for instance. That increases frustration, especially in an emergency. Tape finger cots over all the *call buttons,* and patients can feel their way to the right button. They'll be pleased with the added convenience, and you'll be confident they can reach you when they need you.

—LESLEY GOLDEN, LVN

OVERHEAD SMILE

Despite your best efforts at reassurance, many patients approach a pelvic examination thoroughly tense. To help them relax, tape a "smile face" over the head of the examining table. Then, when the patients spy the happy expression above their heads, they'll invariably laugh, make some comment, and just generally relax a bit—making for an easier, more comfortable examination.

—TONI PILLER, RN

STRAPPED NO MORE

Soft strap restraints used to keep patients from pulling out their I.V.s, na-sogastric tubes, and Foley catheters don't always work well. Some patients wiggle free of the restraints, while others get confused and agitated because their movements are restricted. Sometimes the restraints even inhibit circulation to the patient's fingers.

Instead of straps, pull a stockinette over the patient's hand and up his arm as if it were a sleeve. Then secure the stockinette bottom around the patient's wrist with adhesive tape, being careful not to tape too tightly.

Next, put a sponge ball (the soft kind children play with) into the patient's hand, pull the stockinette back down his arm and over his taped wrist and hand, and tie a knot in the stockinette close to his fingers. Finally, repeat the procedure for the patient's other hand.

With both hands filled, the patient can't get hold of the I.V.s and other tubes. Still, he has freedom of movement—and he can squeeze the balls to exercise his fingers.

—KIMBERLEE A. HULL, CVN

QUICK REPAIR

If your stethoscope's plastic diaphragm breaks or wears out, don't fret. Simply replace it with the bottom cut from a small plastic cup.

—BARBARA C. STENCEL, OBT

MINI VASE

Use the blunt tip of your bandage scissors to snap off the metal ring and rubber stopper of an empty vial. Then you'll have a miniature bud vase—the perfect size for a tiny bouquet of flowers.

—ELEANOR QUIRK, RN

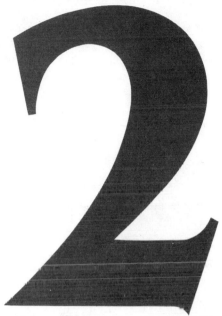

Organize to save time

COLOR-CODED CARDS

To keep instructions for preparing patients for X-ray procedures right at your fingertips, list them on 3x5 cards and keep them in the Kardex. Color-code each index card according to procedure: IVP on a yellow card; gallbladder test on a green card; barium enema on a blue card; and so on. Now, when a procedure is ordered for a patient, just flip through the Kardex until you find the proper color—a great timesaver!

—CHERYL BOEHLY, RN

VITALS UNDER (PLEXI)GLAS

When a number of people are working around a severely injured patient in the emergency department's trauma room, communication of vital signs becomes difficult. To solve this problem, make a large construction-paper chart with columns for time, blood pressure, pulse, and number of I.V. bottles or units of blood. Then cover the chart with Plexiglas and mount it on an easily accessible spot on the trauma room wall.

Using grease pencils, mark the patient's vital signs in their appropriate columns on the chart. This way—at a glance—you can check the patient's most recent vital signs and note any developing trends.

After the initial emergency is over, wipe away the notes with a cloth.

—CALLIE JO SANDQUIST, RN

THE S.P.A.D.E. TECHNIQUE

When you need to make a patient assessment in a hurry and still obtain a maximum amount of information, try the 3-step SPADE technique.

First, determine the patient's status (or progress) in relation to his admitting diagnosis.

Next, assess his general status with SPADE: S—sleep, P—pain, A—activity, D—diet, E—elimination.

Finally, determine his most important request for assistance: "What's the most important thing you'd like to have help with today?"

This abbreviated assessment will help you in reviewing medical orders with doctors and in planning and implementing nursing care.

—E. JANE MEZZANOTTE, RN, MSN

VENOUS EQUIPMENT TRAYED

If you insert subclavian catheters frequently, set up a "Subclavian Tray." A simple, inexpensive plastic utility tray about 8x12 inches (20x30 cm; the kind with a handle) holds all the necessary items:

- a prepackaged catheter
- sterile gloves and towels
- antiseptic skin prep solutions
- gauze sponges
- syringes and needles
- paper tape and adhesive tape
- I.V. tubing and connecting tubing
- antibiotic ointment
- alcohol pads
- a CVP manometer.

—JANEEN HENDRICKS, RN

GRAB BAG

If staff members throw soiled dressings and underpads into patients' wastebaskets rather than discard them in the utility room, correct this situation by installing, near the supply room, a dispenser that holds a roll of large plastic bags. Now, the doctor, housekeeper, or you can easily grab a bag on the way to a patient's room and bag the soiled materials before discarding them. This eliminates odor, contamination, and unsightliness.

—BARBARA LEE, RN

PREVENTIVE CHARTING

Patients can become constipated from the medications they receive for pain control. If this side effect occurs frequently, devise a chart to keep track of patients' bowel patterns and treatment modes. Keep the chart in the front of the Kardex. List patients' names and room numbers in the first column. Head the rest of the columns with the date and divide into three vertical columns—one for each shift.

Use a simple legend: 0 = no bowel movement; B = bowel movement; E = enema; S = suppository. Fill in the chart at the end of each shift. It reminds you to administer treatment before constipation becomes a problem.

—CATHERINE HALEY, RN, BSN

CATHETER KEEPER

If you change catheters on homebound patients, you need to keep several types and sizes of catheters on hand. So use a convenient carrying pouch. Here's how to make it:

Take a piece of canvas (or duck cloth) 72x45 inches (180x113 cm) that has bound edges along its length and cut edges along its width. Fold the canvas in half so the cut edges touch. Sew the cut edges together.

Now fold the canvas in half so the bound edges touch. You've folded the canvas in quarters, so your "pouch" is four pieces thick.

With the bound edges on top, sew a seam down each side. Then stitch seams 5 inches (12.5 cm) apart through all four thicknesses, from top to bottom.

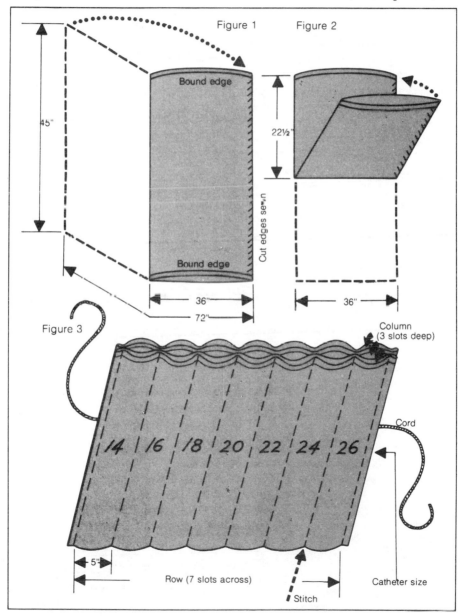

Figure 1   Figure 2

45"

Bound edge

Cut edges sewn

22½"

Bound edge

36"

72"

36"

Figure 3

Column
(3 slots deep)

Cord

14 16 18 20 22 24 26

5"

Row (7 slots across)

Stitch

Catheter size

Your pouch should have 21 slots, in rows of seven across and columns of three deep.

Now take a felt-tip marker and number the first row across according to catheter sizes. Then you can use one column (three slots) for different types of same-sized catheters. For example, in the size-16 column, you can put packages of Teflon catheters in the first slot, plain catheters in the second slot, and silicone catheters in the third slot.

By keeping your catheters in slots, you can easily tell if you're running low. The pouch also keeps the catheter packages from tearing open, which could contaminate the catheters.

If you want to roll up and tie the pouch, sew a 12-inch (30-cm) piece of cord on each side.

—PAM STILGER, RN

TRACTION TREE

The traction room is often cluttered and disorganized. Here's a space-saving, no-cost way to store traction equipment: make a "traction tree." Using extra traction bars, make a trunk, branches, legs, and feet. The trunk is an overhead traction bar, the branches are corner bedpins, the three legs are 18-inch (45-cm) bars, and the feet are short bars of different lengths.

Hang all traction bars on the branches, putting the heaviest bars on the bottom. Because the trunk is slightly off the floor and the legs staggered one above the other, the tree is stable and free-standing. For extra stability, though, attach the tree to a wall with a long traction bar.

—SCOTT GOODRICH

CRASH BOX

Place a "crash box" of emergency supplies on each floor in a place where you can reach it quickly. Each crash box—a clear plastic box about the size of a shoe box—should contain:
- oxygen mask
- oxygen nasal cannula
- instant ice
- airway
- vial of sterile water
- smelling salts
- syringe with needle
- flashlight
- sterile gauze
- tape.

To be sure the boxes are always ready, someone on each shift should check all items, make any necessary replacements, and sign a sheet near the box.

—CAROLYN BIDWELL, RN

MEDICATION INFORMATION

Here's a way to keep track of medications administered on a unit. Post a sheet of paper on the door of the narcotics cabinet. As each narcotic (sedative, pain-reliever, or whatever) is administered, record on the sheet the patient's name, room number, medication, and time it was administered. The sheet provides: (1) quick reference to indicate when a patient received his last medication, (2) a vital information list for the shift report, and (3) a checklist for the narcotic count at the end of each shift.

—A.E. SIMINSKI, RN

PORTABLE POUCHES

Since many nursing home patients use walkers to help them move around, use this device that enables them to carry along such items as tissues, snacks, books, and so forth. Make apron-like carriers from vinyl that fold over the

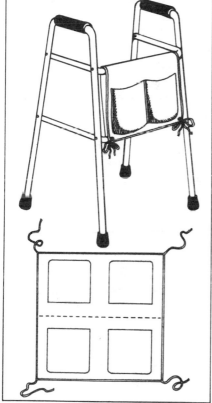

front bar of the walker. These carriers can have four pouches—two in front and two in back—and four strings to anchor them to the front legs of the walker. Besides being handy, these carriers give patients a greater sense of independence.

—JOANNE DORBURY, RN

BOARD AND ROOMS

When hospital personnel need to find a patient, they invariably stop at the nurses' station and ask for his room number. To eliminate these interruptions, construct a board, label it with all the unit's room numbers, and mount the board next to the chart rack, out of public view.

Now when a new patient is admitted, write his name, along with his doctor's, on a piece of tape and attach the tape next to the proper room number. This way the information's available to all personnel who need it, and they can get it themselves—without interrupting you.

—RON YODER, RN

WHAT A DIFFERENCE A TRAY MAKES

Reuse disposable dressing trays as oral hygiene trays; they have three compartments to store all the equipment you need to give patients good mouth care.

In one compartment, put 2x2-inch pieces of gauze. In another, pour your oral cleansing solution; and in the last compartment, store cotton swabs, tongue blades, petroleum jelly, and plastic Kelly forceps. (These forceps are small enough to reach into tiny areas and strong enough to grip the gauze firmly while you're cleaning the patient's mouth.)

The trays help keep supplies together, making mouth care much easier and neater.

—DEBBIE NIEMI, RN

CRASH CARDS

During an emergency you can easily forget the correct medications and procedures to use, in your rush to help your patient.

That's a good reason to list standing-order emergency medications and procedures on cards, and hang the cards in a designated spot on your bulletin board.

Then, if a patient goes into anaphylactic shock, has an insulin reaction, or a cardiac arrest, you can grab the cards for a quick refresher course in emergency nursing. Also color-code emergency drugs for easy identification.

Of course, you should study the cards any chance you get; this way you're prepared before an emergency occurs.

—LARRY ASPLIN, RN

RIGHT IN THE POCKET

To help new nurses become familiar with hospital procedures, print a booklet with information on medication times, surgical preparations, admission and preoperative lab work, and drug and I.V. drip-rate formulas. A 2½x3½-inch (6.3x8.8-cm) booklet fits into a uniform pocket—so the nurses have a convenient reference source near them at all times.

—MARJORIE M. THOMAS, RN

PEARLS OF WISDOM

If you read especially useful suggestions in nursing magazines (call them "pearls"), share them with your entire unit—via a "pearl board."

The pearl board is a large piece of construction paper hung in a central location. Clip the suggestions from the magazine and put them on the board, changing them periodically. For quick reference, save old pearls in a double-pocket folder, also kept on the unit.

—P. GOUGH, RN

FINDING YOURSELF

As you go from one patient room to another, you can easily forget which room you're in if the number's not posted inside. This could cause a delay if you had to call a code or call for help.

To prevent this problem, mark each room's telephone (or some other central object) with the room number on fluorescent tape. Or use a fluorescent marker or crayon to write the number on white paper, then tape it to the phone.

Whichever way you choose, the room number will be clearly visible—even in the dark.

—MARGARET BECKERT, RN

PICTURE THIS

A quick and easy way to measure intake is with a picture chart. Use a paper tray (such as those used to serve meals to patients in isolation) as the background. Cut in half the various sizes of paper

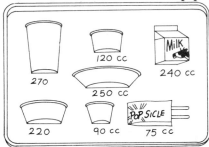

or plastic cups, bowls, cartons, and so forth, and glue them to the tray. Then print the amount of fluids each holds underneath—for example, a carton of milk is 240 cc. Keep this chart on display at the nurses' station. This aid helps you measure intake at a glance when you pick up trays after meals.

—SARAH PETTUS, BSN

NAME THAT PATIENT

In a skilled nursing facility, post a name card at the *head* of each bed, instead of at the foot where it can't readily be seen. Also find out the patient's favorite flower, pet, or hobby and draw an appropriate symbol or paste a picture from a magazine on the card.

The patients will enjoy their decorative identifiers. So will the visitors, housekeepers, and nursing students, who may not know the patients' names and interests.

—BARBARA ROEHRENBECH, RN

TISSUE, TISSUE, EVERYWHERE...

Do you dislike having toilet tissue sitting everywhere and anywhere in a patient's room? And no matter where it is, it's always out of reach when needed.

The solution? Have your maintenance department install toilet tissue holders on an arm of each bedside commode. Then the tissue will always be where it's needed. And even though it's still visible, the tissue's new location seems more appropriate than the windowsill, or the bedside stand, or dresser top, or....

—SANDRA HOLDT, RN

BEDSIDE MATTERS

Do your patients use a bedside commode? To save steps, tie a roll of toilet tissue to one side of the commode with a strip of gauze bandage. On the same side, tie a small plastic bag containing soft pieces of cloth for cleaning patients. Tie another plastic bag for soiled cloths on the other side.

This arrangement not only saves time, but also separates the soiled cloths from the rest of the linen for laundry workers.

—CONNIE DAVIS, RN

COMMUNICATION BOOK

On a busy unit, staff communication can be a real problem—especially between shifts. Sometimes you may not even have time to bring up a question, complaint, or suggestion. So to give everyone a chance to speak up, use a "communication book."

This is a loose-leaf binder in which staff members write their questions—then sign and date their entries. As soon as possible, the head nurse or manager will answer the questions, writing each answer directly below the question, then dating and signing her answer. When indicated, she takes action on the day's complaints or suggestions and notes this, too.

Besides bridging the unit's communication gap, the book can also be educational. Write a brief summary of each inservice meeting and place it in the book for the benefit of those who can't attend.

—DEBORAH GIBSON, RN, MS

SAVE TIME, AHEAD OF TIME

If you frequently have to transfer residents from an intermediate care facility to a hospital or skilled care facility, save time by keeping partially completed transfer sheets for all residents on file at the nurses' station.

Information you can put on the transfer sheet ahead of time includes: name, date of admission, religion, name of closest relative, date of birth, and billing data. Then at transfer time, just add information about the patient's medications and treatments, a description of his diet, a checklist on his ability to perform activities of daily living, and the reason for his transfer.

—JOYCE MARNELL, RN

PATIENT HANG-UPS

Placing a 9½x17½-inch (24x44-cm) cork bulletin board beside each bed on the unit saves time and helps you give better patient care.

For instance, post patient information, such as "limited fluids" or "blood pressure on *right* arm only," on the bulletin board, so nurses on all shifts will know immediately what precautions to take. When a patient is scheduled for a diagnostic procedure the next day, post that information plus whatever preparation is needed ("N.P.O. after

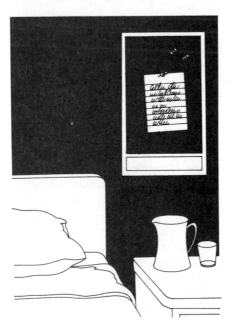

midnight"). And when a patient must go out of his room for an X-ray or physical therapy, put a note on the bulletin board telling where he is.

Using these "patient hang-ups" reduces communication problems among staff, patients, and families.

—JENNY LANGLINAIS, RN

TIPS FOR *TIPS*

Here's how to store helpful tips so you can retrieve them when you need them. Photocopy the tips, then cut and file them in a 3x5-inch file box with alphabetical dividers. If you have a number of tips on one subject—for example, on skin care—make a special divider for that subject and file it under the appropriate letter.

Thanks to this system, your favorite tips are always at your fingertips.

—ANN MILES. RN

GET THE MESSAGE?

A pigeonholed wall cabinet marked with staff members' names works better than a cluttered bulletin board for getting messages and mail to the proper person. The cabinet neatly stores personal coffee mugs, too.

—M.E. GLAVIN, RN

REPORT ORGANIZER

Instead of relying on notes, scribbled on crumpled pieces of paper for change-of-shift reports, use worksheets.

The sheets, kept on a clipboard, should have six columns and room for recording data on eight patients. The column headings can be: name, diagnosis, history; cardiac signs and symptoms; lab data; medication data;

respiratory signs and symptoms; and so on.

Besides making reports more complete and efficient, the worksheets can be used as a reference on nursing and medical rounds.

—DIANE DUBOIS, RN

HOMEMADE FIRST AID

If any of your patients are planning camping trips, you'll do them a service by reminding them to take along a first-aid kit. And it needn't be expensive—they can make it themselves.

Here's what they should do. Take any sturdy container, such as a workman's lunch bucket, and fill it with the following: an antiseptic for killing germs that cause infection; calamine lotion for soothing bites and itches; sterile cotton or cotton-tipped applicators for applying medications; 4x4 gauze pads for large cuts, blisters, or compresses; a 2-inch (5-cm) roll of gauze for bandaging a wound; adhesive tape; an Ace bandage for easing pain and swelling of sprains during the trip to the doctor; scissors; thermometer; tweezers for removing splinters; ammonia capsules for reviving someone who has fainted; and a reputable first-aid guidebook.

Also suggest that they include a list of emergency numbers in their kit, such as: the phone numbers of their family doctor, an alternate doctor, and a relative or neighbor; their hospitalization policy number; and medication prescription numbers.

When they arrive at their vacation site, they can look up the phone numbers of the nearest hospital, a 24-hour or local pharmacy, the police and fire departments, ambulance service, and poison control center, and add these to their list of emergency numbers.

—CATHERINE O'BOYLE, RN

IN THE CAN

A diabetic patient can carry an insulin bottle and two alcohol wipes in a 35-mm film can. The can allows a patient to take his insulin with him wherever he goes, without worrying about leakage or breakage.

—SUE INGRAM, RN

INFO TO GO

Fill a plastic loose-leaf binder with multiple photocopies of patient-teaching handouts on subjects such as low-salt diets, common disease symptoms, precautions for digitalis and anticoagulant use, cleaning respirators, and range-of-motion exercises. Then when a nurse visits a patient, she'll have the handout he needs.

Do handout originals with a felt-tip pen, using large letters. This makes for clear, legible photocopies—a feature welcomed by elderly patients, especially those with poor vision.

—CLAUDIA VEPRASKAS, RN

DOUBLE-DUTY CARD

To reduce duplication of effort when teaching needs of diabetic patients, use a diabetic assessment card.

The front of the card provides space for patient identification.

The back of the card spells out the various responsibilities of staff nurse, inservice instructor, and dietitian.

The staff nurse's duties are to complete the patient assessment; have the patient listen to introductory teaching tapes; reinforce the inservice instructor's teaching; and chart the patient's progress in understanding his diabetic regimen.

The inservice instructor's duties are to provide teaching materials to meet the patient's specific needs; teach the patient individually or in a class; chart the patient's progress in understanding his diabetic regimen; and keep records of the patient's assessment and what he's been taught.

The dietitian's duty is to teach the patient his specific dietary needs.

The diabetic assessment card not only eliminates much duplication of effort, it also ensures that patients' teaching needs *are* being met.

—JENNIFER SPRINGER, RN, BSN

CRUTCH GUIDE

Make a chart that eliminates the trial-and-error approach to adjusting crutches to fit patients. The chart should contain three columns: patient height, proper crutch size, and approximate adjustment for proper crutch length. Then, when you have a patient who is 5 feet 10 inches tall, you look up that height on the chart and see that you should give him an adult-size crutch with the lower bolt placed in the fifth hole from the bottom.

—CATHERINE HALEY, RN

CODE TOOL

During a code, every second counts, so don't waste precious time looking for the proper size endotracheal tube. Have the linen department sew an expandable tube holder (similar to a silverware holder) out of muslin. Make a pocket for each tube and mark the tube size in large numbers on each pocket. Fasten a tie string on each end so you can roll the tube holder into a compact bundle and tie it, ready to use for the next code.

—CHRIS MCSHARRY, RN

NURSING HISTORY HELPER

To help you remember all the pertinent information you need to take a complete, systematic nursing history, use a pocket-sized card as a guide. Here's how to make one.

First, list the categories you wish to include. For example:

- vital statistics
- patient's understanding of illness
- indication of expectations
- social and cultural history
- significant data

Then type these subjects, with questions or specific items to ask the patient about, on both sides of a 5x7 card. Take the card to your hospital's print shop or a local printer and have it reduced in size (to about 3x5) and laminated to withstand the wear and tear of daily use.

The card is handy, easy to use, and lasts for years.

—F. KATE DAVIS, RN

CRASH-CART REVIEW GAME

To help nurses quickly locate any item on the resuscitation crash cart, turn your monthly crash-cart review into a game that helps the nurses learn and remember better.

Before playing the game, divide the nurses into teams of two and give each team a game sheet listing 20 emergency

KNOW YOUR CRASH CART

How fast can you find the following items? Time yourself and see where you rate on the scale below.

- I.V. of 5% dextrose in water, with tubing, tourniquet, needle
- sodium bicarbonate
- airway
- epinephrine
- laryngoscope with #3 blade attached and ready to use
- endotracheal tube #9
- cardiopulmonary resuscitation recording sheet and clipboard
- stylet
- tape
- lidocaine bolus
- tracheotomy tray
- 5-cc syringe
- cardiopulmonary resuscitation board
- Ambu bag
- oxygen mask
- suction machine
- suction kit with catheters
- extra batteries for laryngoscope
- surgical lubricant
- blood pressure cuff and stethoscope

Score:

2 minutes	Super Nurse
2½ minutes	Very Good
3 minutes	Need to review cart
5 minutes	HELP!!!

items. Then, one nurse calls out the items and keeps time, while her partner locates each item on the crash cart.

—CAROLYN LAW, RN

CLIPPED FOR CONVENIENCE

If you're a utilization review nurse, keep your review sheets in a large loose-leaf notebook according to room number and nursing area. Each morning as you check the census to see which patients were discharged or have changed rooms, also see which patients are due for review that day. Then put a paper clip on the bottom of those patients' sheets in the review book. When you complete the review, remove the paper clip.

This way, you can tell at a glance how many reviews have yet to be done. And you have to leaf through the book only once to find out which patients' charts were missing and where you need to go back to do reviews later.

—MARILYN K. DELONG, RN

TRANSFER, PLEASE

If nursing staff members constantly ask for transfers to other shifts or units, track these requests and honor them fairly by using a transfer book.

A staff member who wants a change fills out a request-to-transfer form in the hospital's personnel office. A copy of this form is sent to the nursing office and placed in the transfer book (a large loose-leaf notebook) according to date and position and shift desired. (The book should have a section for RNs, LPNs, nursing assistants, and unit secretaries.)

When a position is available, check the transfer book—before outside applicants are considered. Staff members seeking a transfer should be interviewed as if they were new applicants. If they're not qualified for the position, they're not transferred. But they know they haven't been overlooked.

—PAT YOUNG, RN

FORGET-ME-NOT

Keep a clipboard at the main desk. Write down questions as you think of them. Then before the doctors make rounds, they can check the board and answer your questions.

—SHARON STEVENS, RN

FIRST-AID VEST

As a health professional, why not consider a first-aid vest for your car, rather than the standard first-aid kit? Besides being less cumbersome, the vest will leave your hands free to extricate crash victims, perform cardiopulmonary resuscitation, or give other emergency care.

A good vest to buy is the highly visible blaze-orange kind hunters use. You can put a stethoscope, blood pressure cuff, scissors, penlight, and padded tongue blades in the upper two pockets. Then fill the lower pockets with large trauma dressings, 4x4 gauze pads, and tape.

With a vest like this handy, you'll be able to give quality care—quickly, efficiently, and safely.

—SANDY THORSON, RN

CUT DOWN ON CLUTTER

Tracheostomy patients and those with endotracheal tubes need so much special equipment that their bedside stands are usually cluttered. Use a portable wooden box to accommodate the equipment and have the maintenance department build them to fit on the bedside stands.

The boxes can be 14 inches long, 12 inches wide, and 4½ inches high (35x30x11.3 cm). Divide them into nine compartments to hold gloves, tracheostomy dressings, cotton-tipped ap-

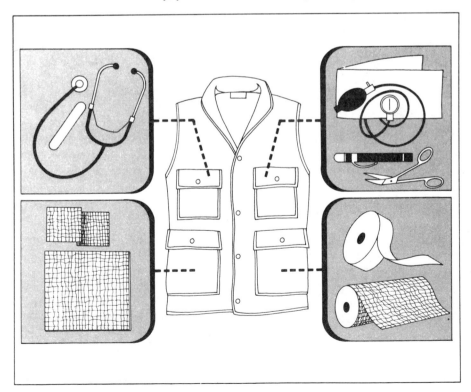

plicators, 4x4s, alcohol wipes, and other equipment. Also, attach a dowel to one side of the box to hold rolls of tape. A drawer, 7 inches long and 1½ inches high (17.5x3.8 cm), on the front of the box can hold alcohol sponges and lubricating jelly.

These boxes are a great boon to bedside neatness and efficiency, and they also show you at a glance what equipment needs to be restocked.

To further cut down on clutter, tape a box of suction catheters to the back of the bed for patients who need suctioning frequently.

—JANE REARDON, RN

ONE GOOD TURN

If many of your patients need to be turned every 2 hours, here's how to give good care, and keep accurate records at the same time.

Put "turn books" by the patients' bedsides. These books are simply three-ring notebooks with columns for recording the time the patient was turned, position of the patient, date, and the initials of the turner.

—MARJORIE KAMTMAN, RN

ALL ON BOARD

Use a magnetic board and magnets in various shapes (squares, stars, circles, and so on) to identify which nurse is caring for which patient.

Write each nurse's name on the board and place a magnet after it. When the desk nurse assigns a patient to a nurse, she puts the same shaped magnet on the patient's chart.

Each nurse can readily see her assignments, and a doctor need only glance at the master board to see which nurse is caring for his patient.

—CALLIE SANDQUIST, RN

COLOR-CODED COLLECTION

Color-code equipment by department for easier location and identification. Say the emergency department chooses red. You then have red stethoscopes, blood pressure cuffs, wheelchairs, airway boxes—even patient records can be red. No longer will you have any question about which equipment is yours and which belongs to another department.

—JEAN CALHOUN, RN
CHERYL WESTBAY, RN

CHECKING IN

Here's how to eliminate unnecessary repetition of calls when emergency team members respond to a *stat* page for a cardiac arrest or multisystem trauma. Next to the trauma room door, mount a Plexiglas board listing doctors and other personnel by their departments: surgery, medicine, anesthesiology, laboratory, and others. When a team member arrives, he checks off his department with a grease pencil attached to the board. You can see at a glance who has arrived and who hasn't.

—NADINE SHLAT, RN

HAMMER HOME

Here's a way to avoid the frustration of being unable to locate a percussion hammer in an emergency department. Make it a *permanent part* of each stretcher. First, attach one end of a 5-foot (150-cm) sash cord chain to the foot of each stretcher; next attach a percussion hammer to the other end of each chain. The length of the chain allows the doctor to move around the stretcher with the hammer. When he's finished using it, he simply slips the hammer and chain under the mattress.

—JUDY ROETHIGER, RN
CHERYL WESTBAY, RN

CLUTTER-ENDING, WALL-SAVING DISPLAY BOARD

Most long-term patients keep their pictures, cards, and mementos on their bedside table. And you must keep moving them—or picking them up off the floor. Mounting anything on the wall with tape, of course, damages the paint.

Here's a solution to these problems: a corkboard 3½ feet (105 cm) high, installed across a major wall in each patient's room. On this, patients enjoy placing family photos, greeting cards, drawings by grandchildren, flags, calendars, wall clocks—anything that can be tacked or hung.

These display boards lend homey individuality to each room, let patients keep their own things, and avoid the annoying problems of wall damage and tabletop clutter.

—DOROTHY HAYFORD, RN
RUTH STRYDER, RN

CUPBOARD I.D.

If your department has many cupboards, locating a particular item can involve a long and annoying search. Here's a way to identify the contents of each cupboard at a glance. Cut the labels from cartons, or the names of products from the literature that accompanies them, and paste these labels on the outside of the door. Now you can quickly find an item just by looking at the labels on the door.

—NAOMI JONES, CRNA

CHARTING CAMPERS' CARE

If you're a camp nurse, record the medications and treatments given campers on separate charts. Then for easy reference, tape the charts to the medication cupboard.

The medication chart should have columns for the campers' names, their medications, and the routes, frequency/time, and day of administration.

The treatment chart should have a column for the campers' names, plus

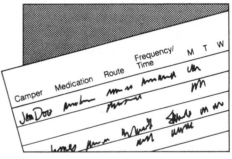

columns for listing their complaints, treatments given, and comments.

These handy forms help you chart efficiently and accurately—even when hordes of campers report in at medication time or when they limp in with bruises and scrapes after sports time.

—SUSAN MAURER, RN

PHOTO FINDER

If elderly patients have trouble finding their rooms, tape a large color photo of the patient's face plus a name card printed in large black letters outside each room. The photo-name cards also help first-time visitors and staff from other departments find specific patients.

—NAN HERNIKL, RN

STEP-SAVER

Ever have to break isolation to get admission items? Or call another nurse to bring the items to the room entrance? The admission procedure can take too much time, too many steps, and too many nurses.

To save time, steps, and nurses, make an admission cart that can be wheeled right to the door. The cart can be an old wooden filing cabinet. Simply add wheels and paint it a bright color. Then you have all the admission items right at the patient's door.

—HEATHER HAY, RN

PLAN WITH PANS

Try to plan ahead for certain types of procedures and examinations. Use three oblong cake pans as an exam tray, eye tray, and ENT tray. Keep all necessary items for these procedures in the appropriate pan.

In one exam tray pan, for instance, keep a flashlight, five tongue blades, reflex hammer, otoscope, ophthalmoscope, tape measure, and safety pin for sensory testing.

The pans fit neatly in supply drawers. When needed, a pan can be taken to the patient's bedside, saving many extra steps in gathering equipment.

—MARY G. ROASAKI, RN

LEAD KEEPER

Lead wires from cardiac monitors often get tangled and are difficult to place on a patient when you're in a hurry. So to keep them straight, attach the leads to a tongue depressor with a piece of tape and label the tape accordingly. Now, when you need to monitor a patient, quickly remove the tongue depressor

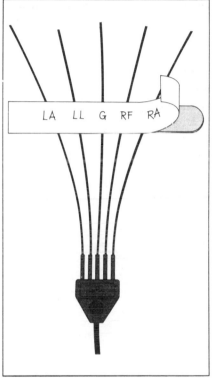

and place the lead on the patient. This technique can eliminate some of the confusion that occurs during emergencies.

—MARY EGGEN, RN

PASS THE TOWEL, PLEASE

Ever have difficulty passing intubation equipment to the doctor, piece by piece?

Gather all the intubation equipment—laryngoscope with blade, endotracheal tube with stylet and inflation syringe attached, oral airway, lubricant, and roller gauze—and wrap it in a disposable sterile towel. Then pass the whole bundle to the doctor with nothing getting lost. This is also handy when the equipment is needed outside the arrest area—the bundle is compact and easily transported.

—YVONNE M. LESIAK, RN

BARIUM ENEMA DILEMMA SOLVED

Ever have to clean up patients who can't retain barium enemas?

Use a "barium enema distress kit," containing a gown, incontinent pads to line the wheelchair, soap, towels, washcloth, small basin, and a few sheets for draping.

—ELIZABETH A. KAYAIAN, SN

SLIPPER HOLDER

Do your patients' slippers seem to play hide-and-seek under their beds? Retrieving these slippers is not only a nuisance for you, but also a danger for

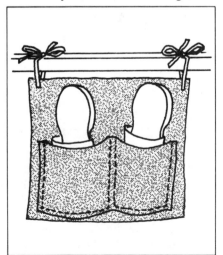

patients, especially the elderly and those with balance problems or limited vision.

Make a slipper holder. All you need is a piece of heavy-duty cloth or canvas, about 16 inches wide and 10 inches (40 x 25 cm) long. Stitch two pockets—about 6 inches wide by 8 inches long (15x20 cm)— to the front of the cloth. Attach strings to the upper corners so the holder can be tied to the side rail or frame of the bed.

—BECKY SCHROEDER, RN

BINDER BENEFITS

If you're a visiting nurse, use loose-leaf binders to maintain patient records.

The benefits of a binder over traditional charting are many. For instance:
• The binder lies flat when opened, and notes can be conveniently and neatly transcribed onto the charts.
• Notes can readily be written on both sides of a page, which cuts the pages per record.
• Preprinted tabs can be attached to the dividers, allowing quick access to record sections.
• Pages can be rearranged easily or added as needed.
• When a binder is full, parts of a patient's record can be removed and filed in a manila envelope, which can then be labeled for easy retrieval.

—LUCILLE GRESS, RN

BEE READY

Here's a way to make life easier for patients who are allergic to bee stings and must carry an anaphylaxis kit. Tell them a plastic travel toothbrush case holds the equipment compactly. Especially convenient for children, the case fits into a back pocket so it can be carried easily outdoors.

To alert others to the patient's prescribed dosage, a prescription label can be attached to the case.

—LINDA DATTOLICO, RN

TIMESAVING CARRY-ALL

Recycle disposable, plastic, self-sealing medication bags that you get from the pharmacy department. Fill them with the items that are often used on your unit but never seem to be on hand. The items may include: prepackaged alcohol and povidone-iodine wipes; lubricant and antiseptic ointment packets; bandages; tourniquet; I.V. labels; and even a pair of nonsterile gloves.

Recycled bags fit nicely into pockets and save time running back and forth for the items.

—PATRICIA MIGU, RN
COLLEEN COPELAND, RN

WHERE ARE THE BAND-AIDS?

If your emergency room has one full wall of drawers, cabinets, counters, and shelves for supplies, number every drawer, shelf, and cabinet. Then make an alphabetical index of all supplies and equipment, listing the numbered location of each.

Then instead of asking, "Where are the Band-Aids?" a person simply looks up "Band-Aids" in the index and heads for the appropriate drawer.

—MARY G. ROASAKI, RN

THE ORGANIZERS

To keep your blood pressure cuffs neatly organized, make a wood box 20 inches (50 cm) long, 10 inches (25 cm) wide,

and 6 inches (15 cm) high. Insert dividers to form eight 5x5-inch (12.5x12.5-cm) cubicles into which your rolled-up cuffs will fit nicely. (Of course, you can tailor the size and number of cubicles as you wish.) The box can be kept in a central location (on a cart, counter, or wall) or moved as needed.

And for handy stethoscope storage,

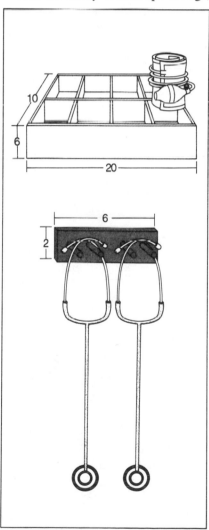

mount two pairs of 3-inch (7.5-cm) dowels on a 2x6-inch (5x15-cm) board attached to the cuff box, or to a wall, cart, or counter end. Then hang your stethoscopes by their earpieces on the dowels.

—TOM CARLSON, RN

ALBUM ENTREE

New patients sometime fear the unknown. To introduce newcomers to the radiation therapy department, take pictures of the treatment machines and of staff members at work. Mount the pictures in a photo album, and add a text that answers patients' most common questions.

The album is a useful aid to patient education. It is easy to design and inexpensive to produce. And the idea can be readily adapted to other hospital departments.

—JUDITH K. STUCKE, RN

ISOLATION REMINDER

When a patient is in isolation, tape a plastic-covered 8½x11-inch (21.3x27.5-

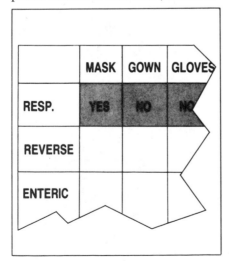

cm) chart to the door of his room. In the first column, list the different types of isolation: respiratory, reverse, enteric, and so on. Across the top of the chart, list equipment you'll be using when working with the patient.

If the patient is in reverse isolation, mark that row with a colored marker; if he's in enteric isolation, mark that row. Then, indicate which equipment requires isolation procedures by writing *yes* or *no* in the square that pertains to the type of isolation and the item.

This door guide reminds you at a glance which procedures you must follow with each patient in isolation.

—PEG KOPPMANN, RN

QUICK FIX FOR STOMA LEAKS

Stoma patients may worry about what to do if their pouches or sites leak. So show them how to prepare an emergency kit. The contents: a pair of underpants, a stoma bag, a small facecloth or premoistened towelettes, and a small, plastic bottle of deodorant.

Men can put all this in a shaving kit; women in a makeup kit. Then the kit can be placed in a glove compartment or desk drawer, where it'll be readily available yet not arouse anyone's curiosity.

—JEAN BOURGELAIS, RN, ET

VOLUNTEER VOUCHER

Volunteer services (such as visits by Reach to Recovery volunteers) can be an important part of patient care, but they seldom get recorded in the patient's chart. What's more, you may have no way to measure the quality of such services. So devise a special "chart" for the volunteers.

Use a gummed label, which the volunteer fills out after visiting the patient and gives to the head nurse, along with a verbal report of the visit. The head nurse can paste the label on the nurses' notes and write a summary of the volunteer's report.

The label includes space for the patient's name, his illness or disability, the date of the volunteer's visit, and the service provided by the volunteer (i.e., prosthesis, exercises, and so on). The label can also have room for comments and for the volunteer's and doctor's signatures.

—MARY E. CORCELIUS, RN

QUICKIE CARD FILE

To keep track of important information you've read, try setting up a quick-reference personal card file.

After you read a pertinent article, list the subject, the source, and the page numbers at the head of a 5x7 note card. Then jot down the article's main points. If you need more cards for the same article, title each one and number them consecutively.

You can also photocopy most charts and tables, and paste them on the cards. Then you can alphabetize the cards with dividers. The cards wear well, don't need much storage space, and can be easily reproduced for your clinical area. They're also great for a quick review.

—LINDA WEITZENKAMP, RN

PICTURE STORY

Even careful documentation of a patient's skin condition doesn't always tell the story as clearly as possible. That's a good reason to include a "Rule of Nines" form—minus the numbers—with your

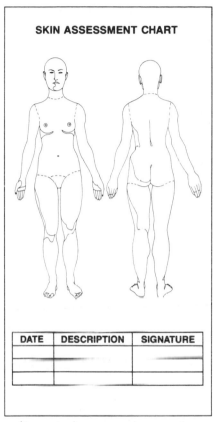

SKIN ASSESSMENT CHART

DATE	DESCRIPTION	SIGNATURE

written notes in your nursing care plan.

Indicate all skin abnormalities on the anatomical form by marking the appropriate areas with red ink. Also write a brief description of the abnormality, including size, appearance, type of wound, and so forth. This gives a picture that's truly worth a thousand words.

—PAT ELSWICK, RN

STEPS TO IMPROVE CRUTCHES

For patients whose hands slip on the smooth surface of crutch handles, cut and affix moleskin adhesive to the handles.

To attach a pocketbook to the crutch, attach a 12-inch (30-cm) dog collar to the crutch handle on the side opposite the injured leg. The collar can be unbuckled and slipped through the handle on any small object your patient wants to carry—like a pocketbook or a portable radio.

—SHIRLEY T. EATON, RN

WHO'S NEXT?

To expedite patient care in an emergency department, number patients' charts in the order they're to be seen. Use 3-inch (7.5-cm) numbers (available at any hardware store) backed with magnetic tape adhesive on one side (available at any art supply or crafts store). Attach the magnetized numbers to the metal portion of the clipboards that hold the charts. They can be easily applied and removed, as the need arises.

—REE MIRAKAMI, RN
CHERYL WESTBAY, RN

LOOK IN THE BOOK

Does your bulletin board get so cluttered with memos, notices, and the like, that important messages often get buried or lost? To be sure all staff members keep up with new directives, procedures, and other such information, put all these memos in a specifically designated three-ring, loose-leaf notebook kept at the nurses' station.

Staff members can quickly check the notebook for new information or easily look up previous notices. At the end of each month, remove the memos and file them where they're still readily available.

—CAROLE S. THOMASSY, RN

FINDING LINES

When patients have multiple I.V. and pressure-monitoring lines, you may have trouble figuring out which line is which.

So color-code the lines. For instance, arterial lines can sport a piece of red tape, pulmonary artery catheter lines may have green tape, central venous pressure lines will bear yellow tape, and each medication line will have a different colored tape marker.

The coding system helps you find the line you need quickly—especially important in an emergency.

—CAROL STEINRUCH, RN

CHECK IT OUT

To make sure you give each patient all the necessary information and handouts, make a checklist.

During the initial interview with each patient, rubber-stamp the inside cover of his folder with a checklist. For an obstetrical patient, for instance, stamp:

___ 1. General information (nutrition, medications, activities during pregnancy, emergency department phone number, and so on)
___ 2. Fee policy
___ 3. Childbirth class information
___ 4. Breast-feeding books and class information
___ 5. Hospital preadmission form
___ 6. Labor and delivery information
___ 7. Insurance forms
___ 8. Last trimester and hospital information.

Then, after each prenatal office visit, check off the information taught or items handed out. This way, you're sure the patient's well informed—on all fronts.

—LINDA J. HAUGEN, RN

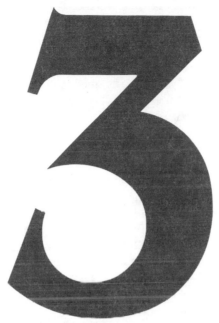

Hot and cold, wet and dry

SOFT TUBE

If you're having trouble passing a Salem sump tube because it's too large for your patient's nares, try running *warm* water over the last 5 to 6 inches (12.5 to 15 cm) of the tube. The water softens the tube, minimizing trauma and discomfort to your patient. Also, water left clinging to the tube helps advance it.

—Deborah Lamb Mechanick, RN

BLOW-DRY SKIN TREATMENT

An extremely obese patient's deep folds of flesh present a real skin-care problem. After his bath, it's difficult to get the skin between these folds completely dry. As a result, the skin may break down.

To solve the problem, use a hair blow-dryer. To be safe, set the dryer on a low speed and always keep it moving. Also test the airflow with your hand to make sure the patient's skin doesn't get too hot.

Besides preventing further skin breakdown, the blow-dry treatment gives the patient's medicated skin creams and powders a chance to work and keeps them from caking together.

—Janet S. Ford, RN

ROLLING PIN RELIEF

Here's a practical and effective way to treat women suffering from back labor. Use two rolling pins—the hollow kind that can be filled with water. Keep one in the placenta freezer and the other at the nurse's station ready to be filled with hot water.

Place a towel on the patient's back

to protect her from the extreme temperature of the rolling pin. Then, with the help of the expectant father, roll one of the pins over the woman's back. The combination of heat or cold and the gentle pressure from the rolling motion seems to give relief.

—RAE K. GRAD, RN

LEAN ON WATER

If a patient's confined to a wheelchair and develops pressure sores from leaning against the armrest for support, reduce the pressure this way. Partially fill a small hot water bottle with water and place it on the armrest. It makes a handy cushion that's just the right size.

—ANN H. PHILLIPS, RN

COOL PAD

Here's a method of applying ice to a patient's perineum after an episiotomy.

First, cut a sanitary pad in half—the short way—and soak the halves in water until saturated. Then take each half and fashion it into a 1-inch (2.5-cm) diameter roll. Next, cover the roll with a 5x5-inch (12.5x12.5-cm) square of plastic kitchen wrap and put it into the freezer.

When the roll's frozen, place one or two Tucks pads on the patient's perineum, put the frozen roll over the Tucks pads, and hold both roll and pad(s) in place with another whole sanitary pad.

—DENISE HOULE, RN

TUBE ON ICE

Ever find yourself in a last-minute rush, looking for a container in which to ice an NG tube before insertion?

Keep a supply of plastic bags and

twist-ties on your dressing cart. Fill a bag with ice, put the tube in it, and fasten the bag with a twist-tie. While the tube is icing, gather the rest of the equipment needed for the procedure. No more rushing!

—SISTER BEVERLY FURTADO, LPN

A TOE HOLD

If a patient needs a warm compress on his toe, use a disposable glove to keep the compress in place and his bed dry. After applying the compress, slip the glove over the patient's toes and lower part of his foot. The glove keeps the compress from getting the bed wet and holds the warmth in longer.

—PAM MILLER, LPN

HOLE IN ONE

Have you ever tried to fill a disposable ice bag—and found you just don't have enough hands? Here's an easy way to do it. Punch out the bottom of a paper cup, fit it in the neck of the ice bag, and use it as a funnel. The ice slides right in.

Warning: Don't leave the cup near your supply of paper cups—you might help yourself to a "bottomless" cup of coffee!

—NOREEN CECHOCKI, RN

IRRIGATING EARS

For ear irrigation, home dental hygiene equipment (the kind with the pulsating stream of water) works better than a syringe ever did. Here's how to use it.

First, make sure the patient's tympanic membrane isn't perforated. Then fill the machine's container with tepid water. Position the patient over a sink or have him hold a basin under his ear. Next, straighten his external ear canal— with children, gently pull the auricle straight back; with adults, pull it back and down.

Then turn the machine on to the lowest pressure setting and aim the water stream directly at the tympanic membrane. If the wax is hard, increase the pressure until the wax begins to break up, then decrease the pressure to finish irrigating the ear. Afterward, tell the patient that if he still feels water in his ear, it will eventually run out.

Finally, sterilize the equipment with a cold sterilizing solution.

—TERRY SCHUMACHER, RN

COOL RELIEF

Itchy skin under a plaster cast is a real problem for orthopedic patients. But a hand-held blow-dryer, set at the cool temperature and aimed at the problem area, readily relieves the itching.

—DEBBIE ALMES, RN

LET IT SLIDE

Filling the ice chamber on a Croupette may be a problem; the ice spills onto the bed or floor. Instead fill a brown paper bag with ice and place it with the open end down into the chamber. The ice easily empties from the bag into the chamber—without a mess.

—MARY BETH FLICKINGER, RN

STIRRUP COMFORT

As any woman knows, those ob/gyn examination-table stirrups can be cold, hard, and uncomfortable.

To minimize this, simply slip a pair of knitted or disposable foam slippers, bottom side up, over the stirrups.

The slippers will certainly help your patients relax. They may even prompt some patients to thank you for your thoughtfulness.

—FAITH KAHLY, RN

SKIN LOTION WARM-UP

Here's one way to avoid applying cold skin lotion to a patient after his bath: Place the lotion bottle, with the cap tightly closed, in the patient's bathwater. As the patient warms up, so does the lotion.

This warm-water treatment also keeps the lotion from thickening.

—GAIL LEW, RN

ICE IN EASY

Unless you have three hands, filling an ice bag can be a messy procedure. Try this ice-bag filler that's inexpensive, washable, long lasting, and—best of all—does the job without the mess.

Have the maintenance staff cut and rivet a piece of metal into the shape of

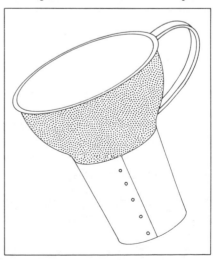

a *bottomless* 6-ounce (180-ml) paper cup. Then have them solder the top of the cup to the bottom of a wide-mouthed metal funnel—the kind used for home canning.

The funnel fits into an ice bag and has a handle for convenient hanging on a hook near the ice machine.

—PHYLLIS BOONE, RN

RELAXING ROUTINE

Ever have difficulty inserting a rectal tube for an enema when the patient's apprehensive? First explain the procedure to the patient, then place a warm, wet cloth against his anal sphincter for a few minutes. This helps the patient relax his sphincter muscle, permitting easy insertion of the well-lubricated tube.

—RENEE BERKE, RN

FRUGAL FUNNELS

Have you ever tried to make an ice bag out of a hot water bottle by stuffing crushed ice into it? Wet and messy, wasn't it? Here's a tidier way. Simply cut the top from an empty half-gallon plastic bleach bottle. Turn it upside down and you have a wide-mouth funnel. Insert the neck of the funnel into the neck of the hot water bottle. The ice will slide in easily, with no mess.

—BROTHER JAMES MARTIN, LPN

Or, to aid in filling ice bags, caps, and collars, cut the large end off a plastic urine specimen bottle and insert it into the neck of the ice bag to make a funnel. You can fill the bag easily without spillage.

—HOLLIS ROBERTS, RN
CYNTHIA HARRISON, RN

PICK FROM THE BUCKET

Here's a way to encourage fluid intake for a patient who's ordered to "force fluids up to 3 liters per day." Ask the food service department to send up a plastic bucket (one for each shift) filled with ice and eight 4-ounce (120-ml) plastic cups. Fill the cups with at least four different kinds of juice and cap with spill-proof lids.

Leave the bucket at the patient's bedside. The patient will look forward to choosing his next drink from his juice bucket. You'll hardly ever have to remind him to take his fluids.

—JANE S. McDERMOTT, RN, BSN

HOMEMADE ICE PACKS

Here's an effective, inexpensive substitute for commercial ice packs.

Simply soak a sponge with water, and place it inside a plastic sandwich bag or zip-lock bag. Then put the bag into a freezer.

One caution: If you use a twist-tie to lock the sandwich bag, be careful that the twist-tie doesn't inflict injury.

—LORRAINE E. LEMUS, RN, BSN

SPRAY THIRST AWAY

Do you have patients on restricted fluid intake? You can help them quench their thirst while using only a small amount of their allotted liquid by using a plastic squeeze bottle with a spray top.

Here's how. At the beginning of your shift, check to see what the patient's allotted amount of fluid is. For example, if he's allowed 50 ml of fluid during the shift, he may wish to use half his allotment in the water spray bottle. Then fill the bottle with 25 ml of water and let the patient spray his mouth as he feels the need. At the end of your shift, measure the remaining amount of water in the bottle. If, for instance, it is 5 ml, you would record an intake of 20 ml from the spray bottle, plus whatever other fluid intake he's had during your shift.

—CHRIS CHRISTGAU, RN

COLD COMFORT

To curb swelling and pain following delivery, tear an opening in one end of a "preemie" disposable diaper and insert a frozen "hot-and-cold pack" between the diaper's plastic and absorbent material. Then apply the diaper's absorbent side to the mother's body.

The hot-and-cold pack stays colder longer, the diaper absorbs any drainage, and the cold can penetrate through the diaper to the patient without giving her freezer burn.

—ADIA F. MEHUS, RN

HOT PACKS A LA SLOW COOKER

Use a slow-cooker crock pot to heat hot packs. Set it to the desired temperature, and you'll have moist hot packs readily available.

—JOANNE E. GERSON, RN

FRUITLESS PRACTICE

With today's high cost of food, using grapefruit and oranges for practicing intramuscular and subcutaneous injections isn't economical.

But here's a suitable substitute: A package of the blue gel that can be frozen and used to cool food in picnic hampers.

Puncture the unfrozen package repeatedly, and it doesn't leak. Pinch it up or spread it for realistic injection practicing. The packages come in various sizes, but the smallest size is most useful.

—JEANNE SORRELL, RN, MS

NO ICE TUBES

If a patient needs a rubber nasogastric tube, don't rush out looking for ice to stiffen the tube. Instead, place a packaged tube in the refrigerator's freezer for about 5 minutes. By the time the patient's prepared, the tube's ready for insertion.

—HERMILA VILLARREAL, RN

JELLY WARM-UP

To help patients relax during sigmoidoscopies and digital exams, warm the lubricating jelly before you apply it. Place the tube upside down in a pitcher of warm water for about 10 minutes. Then when the jelly's applied for the digital exam or sigmoidoscopy, the patient doesn't get as tense as with a cold touch.

—DARLENE ARNSTON, LPN

COOL IT

An elevated temperature is a common problem of postop patients on a surgical unit. Once proper infection-control procedures have been instigated (blood specimen sent to laboratory for culture and sensitivity, antibiotic therapy begun), here's how to lower the patient's temperature while waiting for an aspirin order.

Using a fracture bedpan as a water basin, have the patient place both hands in ice-cold water intermittently for 20 to 30 minutes. This technique has reduced temperatures nearly 2° F. (− 16° C.) in just 30 minutes.

This procedure is ideal for the patient who's sensitive to aspirin; is more comfortable for the patient than alcohol rubdowns; takes less nursing time; and it doesn't require a doctor's order.

—SUE JENNINGS, RN

COLD EGGS

Do you need many sizes and shapes of instant ice packs? For handy, disposable ice cube trays, use old plastic egg cartons. Separate these trays into individual cubes, each in its own egg-shaped container. Then if someone has a lacerated lip or tongue, he can hold the cube to his mouth without freezing his fingers or dripping water on the floor.

—ROSALIND GOLDMAN, RN, SNP

NO-DRIP IRRIGATION

Cancer patients can get shallow excoriated lesions from radiation therapy. Daily irrigation with equal parts of hydrogen peroxide and sterile water can be cold and messy for the patient— when you use traditional irrigating equipment. So try using a sterilized spray bottle instead—the kind used for spray-on glass cleaner. You can deliver an adequate amount of solution, with a minimum of dripping and a maximum of comfort for your patient.

—JOANN TERVENSKI, RN, BS

PAINLESS REMOVAL OF TAR FROM SKIN

Hot tar accidentally splashed on a person's skin can cause painful burns, which can't be treated until the tar has been removed. But when the tar cools it may adhere to the skin, gum up instruments, and if softened with hydrocarbon solvents, merely smear into the wound, causing further pain. Ethyl chloride spray, though it will dissolve the tar, fosters smearing.

To avoid these problems, use a supremely simple method: apply ice to the tar. That hardens the tar into a hard and nonsticky chunk, which can be peeled from the skin without pain.

—DARLA J. SOLDER, RN, ORS

WATER BED FOR THE HEAD

Concerned about the back of a patient's head when he must spend a great deal of time on his back? To relieve discomfort, fill a hot water bottle with 2 cups of water and press out all excess air. With the water pillow under his head, the patient is more comfortable.

—MYRTLE L. LITTLE, RN

REFREEZABLE COLD PACKS

Fill plastic ziplock freezer bags half full with water, remove excess air, and freeze them. They're inexpensive, stay cold longer than the chemical packs, and are available in a variety of sizes for convenience.

—MARGUERITE QUINN, RN

NO MORE COMPLAINTS

If patients complain that they dread the cold speculum during their gynecological examination, here's a way to end the complaints. Keep a jar of warm water in each examining room. Just before the doctor goes into a room, put the speculum in the water. When the doctor's ready to do the vaginal examination, he'll remove the speculum. The warm speculum helps the patient relax, and the water serves as a lubricant to make insertion easier.

—KAREN STARLING, RN, PHN

WARM 'N' READY

To help ensure a patient's comfort during a vaginal examination, warm up those specula.

Put a heating pad into a pillowcase, place both on the examining cart, and turn the pad to a low temperature. Then, set various-sized specula on the pillowcase and cover them with a small towel.

This guarantees your patient a bit more comfort during her examination. It also saves time because the equipment's always at the right temperature whenever you need to use it.

—CATHERINE LAWER, RN

FRESH 'N' SUP

If you don't have time or enough staff to help patients wash their hands and face before meals are served, have the dietary department put an individual disposable towelette on each patient's tray. Patients will then wash themselves, and they'll love the refreshing results. You can also supply towelettes at the bedside for cleansing after bedpan or urinal use.

—ROSEMARY MARTENS, RN

SOOTHING SOLUTION

Here's one way to relieve mouth soreness when patients undergo chemotherapy or radiotherapy. Give them yogurt. Chilled or frozen yogurt soothes the mucous membranes while providing a high-protein snack. (Both regular and diet yogurt contain 8 to 10 grams of protein per 8-ounce container.) Thus, yogurt also helps supply the additional energy patients need when undergoing chemotherapy or radiotherapy.

—CONNIE DANSER, RN

COOL AID

Fill #5 pleated paper cups (the dispenser type) with water, and place in the freezer. When needed, you just remove, fold down the rim extending above the ice, whirl a cloth around the ice end to absorb droplets of water, and apply to the injured part. The paper cup makes it comfortable to hold and easy to move over the injured part, reducing the possibility of ice trauma.

—ANNE SALOKA, RN

HANDY DRYER

Ever have a problem drying empty hot water bottles and ice bags? A simple help is a wire coat hanger. Hang a hot water bottle upside down by placing the hanger hook through the hole in the bottom of hot water bottle.

To dry ice bags, pull down on the bottom of the coat hanger, then bend elongated hanger in half. Slip the ice cap over the end of the bent portion of the hanger.

—MARILYN A. METKER, RN

ICE BAGS THAT FIT

Need a good ice pack for hard-to-cover areas such as your patient's knee, cast, or forehead? Use the plastic bag that holds the supplies issued to each patient on admission.

Fill one fourth to one third of the bag

with ice and secure it with a heavy rubber band. Then turn the remaining portion of the bag inside out—over the ice-filled part—and pull the drawstring or fasten with another rubber band. You'll have an ice pack that's double thick, moldable, and usually just the right fit.
—DAVEEN MCCLURE, RN

OTHER PLASTER PROBLEMS
Always use cold water for easy removal of plaster from patients and instruments after a cast has been applied. If you get plaster on your uniform, let the plaster dry, then brush it off.

Since working with plaster can dry your hands, keep a bottle of hand lotion nearby and use it frequently.

Let mothers soak the serial casts off their babies. And add a little vinegar to the water to aid removal of the casts.
—ELSIE HAJDICS, RN

GONE FISHING
Have you ever tried to apply an ice pack to a small child's hurt finger? Not an easy job, at best. Next time, instead of struggling, turn the ice treatment into a game.

Fill a plastic mug with ice and water and challenge the child to get the ice out of the mug. While he's fishing for the ice, the icy cold water will decrease swelling and pain. He'll forget about his sore finger, and you can dry his tears.
—CATHY PARKER, LPN

PRETTY COOL SOLUTION
FOR SEVERAL PROBLEMS
There's a simple, enjoyable way to solve certain problems: ease bleeding of cut lips or tongue of crying children...ease

swelling gums of cranky oldsters after dental procedures...administer fluids to patients of any age apt to vomit. It's a *Popsicle*.

It's a valuable item, especially for children, when the doctor wants to start certain patients on fluids by mouth, as after acute gastroenteritis or surgery, or when ordinary fluids are apt to precipitate vomiting. And, needless to say, patients almost invariably enjoy the cold treat.
—ADELAIDE ROSEN, RN

ICE SEALING
To improvise an ice pack, try using the kitchen appliance that seals a meal into a plastic bag. Fill a large-size bag with ice and seal it. Apply this pack to the affected area. The ice will melt, but the pack remains cool. And no leakage.

Place the bag of water in the freezer and you have an ice pack ready for the next injury. You can make a few in various sizes and keep them in the freezer at the hospital for your patients.
—SHERRI SENER, RN, BSN

MORE PLEASING BY
FREEZING
When a patient has trouble swallowing, because of throat surgery or a hampered gag reflex resulting from a stroke, taking liquids may be a problem. But freezing liquids is helpful. Patients can swallow high-protein and high-calorie items such as Sustacal, milk shakes, and eggnog much more easily when they're in a semisolid state. Another advantage: freezing makes less-desirable liquids more palatable.
—BARBARA D. MIZENKO, RN

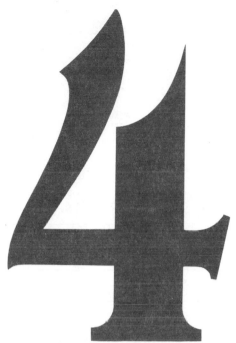

I.V. therapy made easier

A PULL TOOL
To remove a stubborn needle from I.V. tubing or a syringe, wrap one end of some Penrose drain tubing around the I.V. needle's hub and the other end around its adapter. As you twist in opposite directions, the Penrose tubing "grabs" the line to help you pull out the needle.

—NANCY PEREZ DIATIMA, RN

TENDER GLOVING CARE
If you use a heparin lock, instead of an I.V. line, to keep a patient's vein open, the lock and the dressing may get wet when the patient takes a shower. This will loosen the tape securing the I.V. needle, causing the needle to slip out.

Instead, keep the lock and dressing dry with an inexpensive, nonsterile examination glove. After cutting the fingers off the glove, slip it over the patient's arm. Fit the glove neatly over the lock and dressing, then wind hypoallergenic tape around the glove ends to seal the glove and affix it to the patient's arm.

Thanks to the glove, patients can take showers without worrying. And you don't have to waste time (and patients' money) reinserting I.V. needles and starting new heparin locks.

— SARA M. KERESTER, RN

I.V. INFORMATION
When checking I.V.s use *one* master chart—just for I.V. information. The chart should have columns for the patient's name, age, room number, diag-

nosis, I.V. flow rate, type of solution, and amount left from the previous shift.

At the end of the shift, or during a slow period, transcribe the information onto the individual patient charts.

The master chart tells you at a glance which patients will need a new I.V. bag hung, and when. It saves time and steps.

—LINDA T. DEAN, RN

TAPE PUT-ON AND TAKE-OFFS

When taping a patient's I.V. needle to his arm, wipe the sticky underside of the tape (the section that will be next to his skin, not the ends that will attach to the armboard) with a cotton ball. Pieces of cotton stick to the tape, making a soft, nonirritating surface that can easily—and painlessly—be removed from the patient's skin.

—JEANINE WHITAKER, RN

THE LIGHT TOUCH

If you suspect I.V. infiltration in a patient with difficult veins, turn on a flashlight and hold it against his skin, directly over the suspicious site.

If I.V. fluid has infiltrated into the tissue, the beam will highlight the size of the infiltration. If no fluid has infiltrated, only a small halo will appear around the flashlight.

Using this trick can save you from having to do extra checks. Then, if necessary, you can stop the I.V. before the infiltration gets worse.

—BETTY WOODFIN, RN

PUT THE PRESSURE ON

If you have to insert an I.V. in the dorsum of a patient's hand and can't find

his veins, simplify the search. Apply a blood pressure cuff to the patient's arm below the elbow. Then pump the

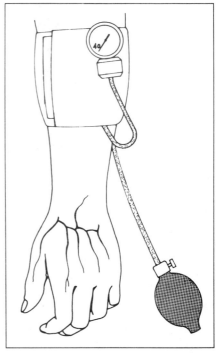

cuff to 40 mm Hg and wait about 2 minutes for the small veins to appear on the hand.

The blood pressure cuff helps you locate veins better than a conventional tourniquet.

—LARRY K. KING, RN

TOWEL TRICK

Here's an effective way for students to practice changing I.V. tubing. Half fill a small, plastic trash bag with rolled-up towels, and knot the bag at the top. Then roll the bag into the shape of an arm and insert a catheter through a single thickness of plastic and into a towel. Attach the catheter to I.V. tubing and attach the tubing to an I.V. bag filled with water.

Now students can practice changing and taping the tubing and learn how to regulate the flow clamp. What's more, they don't make a mess because the towels absorb the water.

—LINDA SCHAFFER NEWMAN, RN

GETTING IT PEGGED

Don't waste time sorting through containers of I.V. additives and preparing I.V.s for patients. Instead, have the maintenance department make a pegboard with long hooks to hang in the medicine room. Then, the pharmacist can prepare the additives, hang them on the hooks in the proper series order, and mark each hook with the patient's room number. Besides saving time, it also eliminates errors.

ESPIRANZA CASTELLANOS, RN

GENTLE REMINDER

To remind a patient not to bend his hand or wrist when he has an I.V. inserted, try this. Cover a peripad with a washcloth, and tape the covered peripad to the patient's palm and forearm. This makes a soft, nonbulky armboard—a subtle reminder to the patient to keep his wrist or hand straight.

—LOU ANN JEFFRIES, RN

MAKING CONNECTIONS

When giving I.V. medication via a volume-control set, try securing the needle in the primary line's secondary port this way:

Cut a 3-inch (7.5-cm) piece of 2-inch-wide (5-cm) adhesive tape. Fold over each end ½ inch (1.2 cm) to make double-thick, nonadhesive flaps for easy removal. After inserting the needle into the port, center the tape (adhesive side up) under the connection, bring the tape ends up, and secure them to each other.

To remove the needle from the port, simply pull the flaps apart.

—JOY TAUROZZI, RN

I.V. CHECK CHART

Have you ever gone to check a patient's I.V. intake only to find the Kardex in use? Do you find medicine cards too time-consuming to maintain? Then, perhaps you'll like an I.V. chart.

It's easily made by cutting two pieces of cardboard to a size suitable for the number of patients' I.V.s you want to list, say 10 by 12 inches (25 by 30 cm) with enough room for eight patients. Cover both pieces of cardboard with attractive Con-Tact paper and cut the required number of holes about 2 by 3

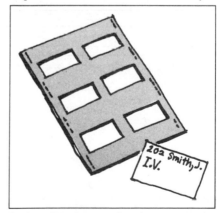

inches (5 by 7.5 cm) in one piece. Using staples, tape, or paste, fasten the cut-out cardboard piece on top of the other, leaving space at the sides to insert small pieces of paper to show through the cutouts.

Each patient's name, room number, and I.V. is put on a slip of paper. If a patient has several I.V.s, note each I.V. on a separate slip.

When a new I.V. is hung, place this slip in front of the old one. Thus, a quick glance at the chart tells what I.V. each patient has running at any specific time.

—NANCY L. SCANLAN, RN

QUICK CHECK FOR I.V.S

When you have several patients receiving I.V. fluids, a quick way to check on the absorption rate is to attach a piece of adhesive tape lengthwise to each bottle. At the top of the tape, mark the time the solution was hung. At the bottom of the tape, mark the time the solution should be absorbed. Midway

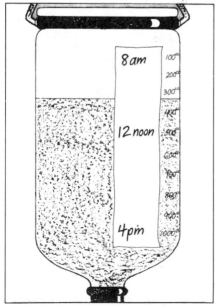

between these two labels, mark the time when half the amount of the solution should be absorbed. With these mark-

ings, you'll be able to see at a glance whether the solutions are being absorbed on schedule.

—SYLVIA E. PLATT, RN

EDEMA DILEMMA

Here's a way to insert an arterial or I.V. line into a patient's edematous arm.

Elevate the patient's arm and wrap it—from his hand to his shoulder—with an elastic bandage. Suspend the arm from an I.V. pole with another elastic bandage for 10 minutes. The edema will disperse and the forearm will return to normal size.

Then, with the sterile field and equipment prepared, quickly lower the patient's arm and unwrap his hand and lower forearm. Palpate the artery or vein, and you can insert the needle easily.

—LT. MELANIE THORNTON, ANC

BOXED BOARDS

If an I.V. armboard isn't available when you need one, just tape a washcloth or small towel around the empty I.V. tubing box and use that instead. The long, narrow box makes an excellent temporary I.V. armboard and saves you the time of looking for the real thing.

—CAROL KENCK CRISPIN, RN, MEd

SHOWER SLEEVE

The problem: How to keep an I.V. from getting soaked and becoming dislodged when the patient takes a shower.

The solution? Cover his arm with a long plastic bag that holds disposable drinking cups. Cut off both ends of the bag, slip it over his arm, and tape it at the wrist and upper arm with nonallergenic tape. The I.V. stays dry, and your patient can enjoy his shower.

—SUSAN FREER, RN

I.V. STOP SIGN

When an I.V. is to be discontinued after the patient has absorbed all the fluid, tape a Band-Aid and a packaged alcohol swab on the I.V. bottle. Not only will this save time (no running to get these items when the I.V. stops), but it confirms at a glance the discontinue order.

—PATRICIA WILSON, RN

NOW, BREATHE DEEPLY

Before inserting an I.V. needle, have your patient practice a simple breathing exercise: Inhale deeply through the nose and exhale slowly through the lips. Then, as you insert the needle, ask him to repeat this breathing technique. This will make him less tense, so the venipuncture will be smoother and less painful.

—SANDRA G. ROSS, RN

IMPROVISED ARMBOARD

When you start an I.V. in a patient's lower forearm, wrist, or back of the hand, you may want to use something other than a conventional armboard for immobilization. An aluminum forearm splint works fine. It's comfortable, lightweight, and small enough to fit comfortably.

—DARLENE LAINCHBURY, RN

QUICK TRICK FOR I.V.S

When the I.V. runs dry and you need to hang another bottle but air is in the tubing, here's a quick way to change bottles without breaking a closed system or introducing a needle into it. First, slide the drop regulator down the tubing as far as possible (usually to the Y site) and close it. Remove the empty bottle and hang the new one. Squeeze the drip chamber to get fluid into it.

Then grasp the tubing just above the drop regulator, using your thumb and a hard object (such as your closed scissors or a pen) to compress it. Move your hand up the tubing, causing the fluid to push the air into the drip chamber. (Note: Your hand will slide easily if you first wet the tubing with an alcohol sponge.) Then release your grasp and turn on the I.V.

—P. SEIBEL, RN

A GAUZE GOODY

In I.V. therapy, armboards may present two problems: the adhesive tape used to anchor the board might irritate the skin; and, although multiple pieces of tape are used, the board may still be unsteady.

A solution is to place the armboard in the appropriate position and wrap 4-inch (10-cm) gauze around the arm and board, securing the gauze with one piece of tape not in contact with the skin.

Besides saving the patient from tape irritation, the stability is particularly valuable when a patient is agitated or has to be moved.

—MICHELE A. CAWLEY, RN, MN

I.V. INDICATOR

The self-adhering peelback I.V. labels can save you time and effort. Here's one way to use them.

When you start an I.V., peel off the

back of the right-hand side of the label and attach it to the I.V. bottle so the label markings align with those on the bottle. At the top of the label, mark the time the I.V. was started. This way, the label serves as a check on the absorption rate.

When the solution has been absorbed, remove the label, peel off the rest of the backing, and stick the label on the patient's chart. Besides the patient's name, the date, and room number, the label has space to write the fluids and medications administered. You can then complete the label information, adding when the I.V. was discontinued, the bottle number, rate of flow, and your signature. This completes the patient's record, eliminating the need for an I.V. stamp.

Labels are available for both 500-ml and 1,000-ml bottles.

—MARGARET E. DUNN, RN

CLEAN AND DRY

When a patient with an I.V. line in his hand or wrist wants to take a sponge bath, have him put on a sterile glove. The glove extends to about the mid-forearm, keeping the I.V. site clean and dry during his bath.

—CHERRI BRIGHT CRONEN, RN

WEIGHT UNTIL THE CALM

The thrashing and pulling of confused, combative patients sometimes necessitates restarting I.V.s several times. So, after establishing an I.V., place a 5-pound (2.2-kg) sandbag under a standard armboard. Then wrap the sandbag, armboard, and arm with an Ace bandage. The weight of the sandbag, which can be varied as needed, keeps the arm immobile.

—ANN HENSLEY, LPN

LESS MESS LESSON

When nursing students practice using I.V. equipment with emesis basins to collect the solution, many times the tubing slips and the solution runs onto the floor, making a sticky mess. Solve this problem by having them use an empty, used I.V. bag to represent the patient's vein and collect the solution.

Just insert the needle from the tubing of the practice bag into the medication port of the empty I.V. bag. The tubing port of the empty bag can be clamped with a hemostat or plugged with an I.V. needle protector (which must be taped in place). Students can then regulate I.V. flow, check for backflow, remove air from the tubing, administer medications by I.V. push and piggyback, change I.V. tubing, and practice other I.V. skills with realistic results—and no mess.

—ROSEMARY FISCHER, RN

GET A GOOD GRIP

Changing I.V. tubing isn't always easy—especially when the connection to the catheter's been forced or "glued" shut with blood. In fact, if you try to pinch the old tubing away or use a hemostat to pull it, you could dislodge the catheter.

A better method is to wear rubber gloves. This gives you a better grip on the tubing, and usually you'll be able to pull it away without dislodging the catheter.

—DAVID VLAHOV, RN, BSN

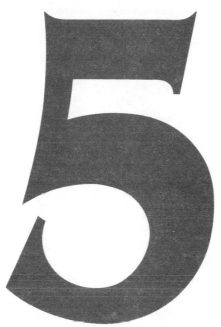

Improving drug administration

MASTERING THE MIX

Ever have to show diabetic patients how to draw the right amounts of regular and NPH insulin into the same syringe without mixing the different insulins in their bottles? To help patients practice this, use sterile water and red food coloring to simulate the two kinds of insulins.

First, inject 10 ml of water into an empty insulin vial and label it "regular insulin." Then, inject 1 ml of red food coloring into a second vial, labeling it "NPH insulin."

When the patient draws the two "insulins" from the vials into a syringe, the color will tell him how accurately he's measured the correct amounts of "regular" and "NPH" insulin. Also, any food coloring in the vial of water or cloudiness in the food coloring vial will show that he's mixed the insulins the wrong way.

—NANCY SCHLOSSBERG, RN

SPECIAL LIST

Before distributing medications from the unit-dose cart, quickly thumb through the medication sheets and make a list of other-than-routine administration times. Also list patients receiving hourly doses of a particular medication as well as patients receiving I.V. medications. Then use this list to ensure giving all medications at the time ordered.

—ELLEN LUDIN, RN

PICK YOUR FLAVOR

If your patient dislikes milk of magnesia's taste, try adding a little of the flavoring designed for liquid dietary supplements. Some supplements offer pecan, cherry, lemon, orange, and strawberry flavors.

Whichever flavor your patient chooses, chances are it'll help his medicine go down easier—and with no unpleasant aftertaste.

—JOCELYN MORITZ, RN

DOUBLE CHECK ON DRUGS

To prevent drug interactions, you need to know what medications a patient is taking when he's admitted to the hospital and where those medications are being kept during his hospitalization. Recording this information on the back of the patient's Kardex works well. The information is right at your fingertips whenever it's needed.

—DORIS SEDBERRY, LVN

MEDICATION REFRIGERATION

Store aluminum hydroxide (Amphojel) in the refrigerator. When the medication's cool, it doesn't leave a chalky sensation in the patient's mouth. Also, the patient seems more aware of the drug's cool temperature than of its unpleasant flavor.

—PENNY PICA, RN

BAGS ARE BETTER

To cover an application of nitroglycerin paste on a patient's arm, use a plastic sandwich bag instead of plastic wrap. With its bottom cut off, the bag fits over most arms like a sleeve and stays secure with just a bit of tape. Best of all, it doesn't snarl as easily as plastic wrap.

—SARA WISTER, RN

SYRINGE VERSUS SPOON

Oral antibiotics are prescribed for many of the babies brought to an emergency department. You usually administer the first dose, using a syringe to squirt the medication into the baby's mouth, then give the baby's mother the prescription for the remaining doses. But if the baby needs a second dose during the night—before the mother can get to a pharmacy—give her a single dose to take home.

A disposable syringe makes an ideal container for a single dose of oral medication. When you give the initial dose, show the mother how to use the syringe safely.

—E. ROGERS, RN

SLIDE SHOW

Here's a quick and inexpensive way to teach patients to identify their nonliquid medications: Just slide individual dose packs into the slots of a clear plastic holder for 35-mm slides.

The dose packs have the name and strength of the drug printed on the back, so patients can get this information on one side and then flip to the other side to see what the medication looks like. If dose packs aren't available, you can tape the pills onto the front of a label and write the name and dosage on the back.

—CARLENE GRIM, RN, MSN

TWO BANDS BETTER THAN ONE

To prevent medication errors, suggest that all patients with medication allergies wear identification different from the rest of the hospital population.

For instance, allergic patients could wear two wristbands: the regular identification band worn by all patients and another specifying the patient's allergy. Or, they could wear just one wristband in red (or green) to distinguish it from those worn by other patients.

Although some allergic patients have their own "Medic-Alert" bracelets or necklaces, many don't. So a hospital-wide system of identifying them is a good idea.

—KAREN L. POLINSKI, RN, BSN

CAPS OFF

If you're caring for arthritic or elderly patients who skip medications because they can't remove child-proof caps from medicine bottles, these tips may help.

Many child-proof caps have two parts: an inner part that screws onto the bottle, and a revolving outer part that provides the safety feature. Dig out the inner part, discard the outer, then use the inner part to cap the bottle. The patient will now be able to open the bottle easily.

Better yet, you can avoid this whole problem by suggesting that your patients request regular caps for the bottles the next time they get their prescriptions filled.

Of course, if children are present in the home, you'll want to disregard these tips.

—LORRAINE CASTELLINO, RN

KEEP IN GOOD SPIRITS

Allowing one or two family members to stay with an anxious patient in the emergency department helps calm the patient. But sometimes a family member becomes ill or faints. To handle such "visiting emergencies," keep two ampules of spirits of ammonia on double-backed tape within easy reach in each cubicle. The faster you revive the visiting patients, the sooner you can get back to the "real" patients.

—MARY KENNEDY EGGEN, RN

WHAT'S THE WORD?

When administering antibiotics through a heparin lock, do you ever have trouble remembering each step? Use this acronym to help remember the procedure:

*S*aline, 2 ml—to clear the lock
*A*ntibiotic—through the lock
*S*aline, 2 ml—again, to clear the lock
*H*eparin—to keep the lock patent.

"SASH" works fine, but you can make up your own reminder based on the procedure used at the hospital where you work.

—SHIRLEY COSTANZA, RN

TWIST-OFF CAP OFF

If you're ever stuck with a hard-to-open pour-bottle of liquid medication, try wrapping any flat piece of rubber 1½ times around the cap. You'll find that the cap will unscrew with just a gentle twist.

Rubber tourniquets are ideal.

—DIANE PUTA, RN

QUICK DISSOLVE

If you have to administer tablets or capsules through a nasogastric tube because no liquid replacements are available, remember that the medication will dissolve more rapidly and completely in *warm* water. And since less warm water is needed to dissolve the medication, a patient on fluid restriction won't get too much liquid.

—BARBARA A. MATHEUS, RN, BSN

A SPEEDY, SAFE WAY TO IDENTIFY DRUGS FOR CARDIAC ARREST

Coping with cardiac arrest requires various drugs in syringes—quickly identifiable. And there's always a risk they might get mixed up. In some hospitals, the syringes are labeled by someone writing directly on the barrel with pencil or felt pen. Here's a way to do it quickly—and safely.

Take ½-inch-wide (1.2-cm) adhesive tape. On it write the names and dosages of various drugs needed in an emergency. Then cut the tape into separate labels and stick them on a sheet of clean X-ray film. This doesn't affect their adhesive property.

Keep the film and attached tape strips on the cardiac emergency cart. Then, in arrest, merely pull off the right label and stick it on the syringe.

This not only saves time—it always assures having a record of the drugs actually used during the resuscitation. It also simplifies figuring what drugs to replace afterwards.

—CATHERINE A. BADEN, RN, MS

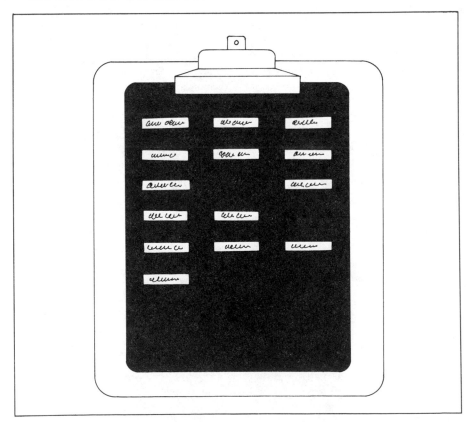

P.R.N. LIST

Ever have trouble remembering to give p.r.n. medications? Just keep a p.r.n. list on the medication cart. The list should have columns for time of request, patient's name, medication requested, and medication given. Never fill in the last column until *after* you've given the medication.

Now you have a fast, accurate way to check the medications given if the narcotics count is ever off at the end of the day. And patients get faster service, too.

—VIVIAN HALL, RN

BOTTLE CLIP

A simple, inexpensive broom clip holder helps a one-handed diabetic prepare his insulin independently.

The clip, available in most hardware stores, holds a standard-size insulin bottle securely and can be mounted on any convenient surface with a single screw. An easy-to-reach kitchen cabinet shelf usually works well. (Of course, the clip shouldn't interfere with the cabinet door closing.)

—JUNE B. JACKSON, OTR

SINGLE FILE

If you give many medications by I.V. push, you know these medications require various amounts and kinds of diluent and can be given safely at various speeds. However, if you can't take the time to read the detailed literature each time you give a medication, solve the problem with a recipe box. Keep a file card for each medication in alphabetical order. Each card should include information about dilutions, rates for pushing, alternate names, side effects, contraindications, and other pertinent information. This is a valuable tool for new nurses, especially in emergencies.

—RUTH L. HORMAN, RN

SHOE BOX/PILL BOX

If a blind patient is taking a variety of medications, all in pill form, and wants to take them by himself, use this system: Using letters cut from sandpaper, label seven envelopes with the days of the week. Place the pills in small zip-lock plastic bags labeled with sandpaper numbers, according to the time the pills are to be taken. Then, place the bags inside the envelopes, and file the envelopes in a shoe box within the patient's reach.

At the beginning of each day, the patient simply pulls the first envelope from the box, "reads" the numbers on the plastic bags with his fingers, and takes his pills at the designated hours.

This system not only gives the patient a feeling of independence, but it also gives you an accurate way to tell whether he's taken all of his pills.

—BARBARA BOLES, RN

RIGHT SIDE UP—AND DOWN

Do your patients on twice-daily medications have trouble remembering whether they've taken their morning or evening dose? Here's a way to help them keep track.

Tell them to mark the top of the medication container "a.m." and the bottom "p.m." Then, as soon as they've taken the medication, they can turn the container to show the time for the next dose. Later, if they've forgotten whether

63

they took their medicine that morning, they can simply look at the container. If it shows "p.m.," they know they took the morning dose.

—WILHEMINA K. PATTERSON, RN

IN THE CARDS

So many new chemotherapeutic agents are being prescribed for cancer patients, you can be hard pressed to keep up to date. Gather the information about dosage, route of administration, side effects, and specific nursing implications (if any) for each new agent prescribed. Then print or type this information on a 3x5 card and enclose it in plastic to protect it. Keep these cards on the Kardex for easy access and quick reference.

—CAROLE W. SWEENEY, RN

DOWN THE STRAW

If a patient needs a nitroglycerin tablet but can't place the tablet himself—or even lift his tongue to let you place it— a drinking straw can help.

Just put one end of the straw under his tongue and drop the pill down the straw. Pull the straw back slightly, then lift the tongue with the straw to make sure the tablet's properly positioned. If everything checks out, remove the straw.

—ZOE MARGOLIS, RN, BS

SUN WATCH

Patients on phenothiazines (Thorazine, Chlorpromazine, Promacid, and so forth) often become photosensitive. To remind you to caution the patients about the drugs' side effects, attach a small yellow card to the patient's Kardex record. On it, draw a picture of the sun and write the message "WATCH FOR THE SUN."

Now you'll remember to teach these patients how to guard against sunburn.

—LA DONNA TATE, RN

MED UPDATE

Instead of constantly checking through the medications on your unit to keep track of expiration dates, record them on your calendar. Write the name of each drug on the date of its expiration. Then, at the beginning of each month, check the calendar to see which medications should be returned to the pharmacy for replacement.

—KATHY DiCARLO-BARBATO, RN

POP TOP PROTECTION

When giving medications, how often do you find yourself in such a hurry that you pop the top off an ampule without using gauze or cotton to protect your fingers? A solution is to carry a nipple in your pocket. Just place the nipple over the ampule and snap the top off—no more nicked or cut fingers. You can easily clean the nipple with alcohol to prevent cross-contamination.

—HAROLD L. HARDGRAVE, LVN

GOOD DEAL OF INFORMATION

Many patients are unfamiliar with side effects of their prescribed medications. Give the patient an index card listing the name of the medication, possible side effects, and what the medication does. Of course, write this in terms the patient will understand. Preparing these cards helps you keep up on pharmacology, and the patients appreciate the extra care.

—CHRISTINE A. PRONZO, RN

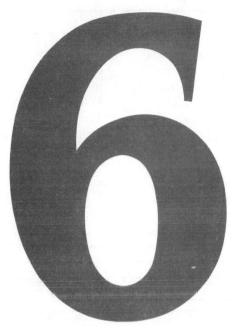

Caring for adult patients

SAY IT WITH FLOWERS

If you ever have to explain collateral circulation to a myocardial infarction patient and his family, compare your patient's injured vessel to the stem of a plant that's been accidentally broken off. When placed in a glass of water and given some time and care, the stem will sprout new roots. So, too, the patient's heart with proper care and rest will sprout new vessels.

Not only does this explanation bring a difficult subject into clearer focus, but it also gives the patient some much-needed hope for recovery.

—DIANA MCLEOD, RN

SAVE THE SKIN

Giving *total* skin care to patients with Sengstaken-Blakemore tubes starts with a football helmet. Have these patients wear a helmet, and instead of taping the tube to the patient's skin, tape it to the helmet's mouth protector. Then when traction is released, give skin care to the patient's back, shoulders, and buttocks as needed. And after you remove the helmet, massage the back of his head, ears, and neck.

—MARGERY LEBEL, RN, CCRN

PREVENTIVE MAINTENANCE

When catheterizing a patient, here's how to prevent the sterile field from folding back on itself after you've carefully spread it out.

Roll two pieces of tape into rings with the sticky side out. Unpackage—but don't unfold—the sterile field, and place it between the patient's legs. Put one piece of tape on what will be the underside corner of the field that you'll be opening toward you. Pull open the field, and secure the taped corner on the thigh (for a man), or sheet (for a woman). With the other tape ring, do the same on the corner that opens away from you.

This little bit of tape is a great preventive maintenance tool—especially when the patient won't or can't remain still.

—WARREN G. PATITZ, RN

PAINLESS TAPING

Teaching patients or their families how to dress and redress wounds on hairy areas of the body can be a problem, because the tape sticks to and pulls the patient's hair when it's removed. Shaving the area helps, but the tape still gets caught on some of the hair. Solve the problem with pink hairdressing tape. It keeps dressings as secure as regular tape, but it lifts off easily and with less discomfort to the patient.

—NANCY E. DIRUBBA, RN, FNP

PUT A LID ON IT

Some bedridden patients spill more than they drink whenever they use a cup or glass. So ask their families to bring in an empty pint-size jar with a screw-on lid. (A mayonnaise jar is a good example.)

With a nail that has about the same diameter as a straw, punch a hole in the middle of the lid. Then pour the liquid into the jar, screw on the lid, and put a straw through the hole. The patient can drink away—and not spill anymore.

—DEANN MEYERS, RN

HOOK THE BAG

Have trouble ambulating a Foley catheter patient by yourself? Ask a hospital maintenance man to put a hook on the lower part of each movable I.V. pole. This hook holds the catheter bag more securely than a pin on the patient's clothing. Also, the patient can hold on to the I.V. pole for stability—and you can ambulate him by yourself.

One caution: Make sure the catheter tubing doesn't hang low between the patient and pole. Otherwise, the tubing could get caught under the pole's wheels.

—CHARLENE FORVERY, LPN

NO MORE NUMBNESS

When treating a patient's sore throat with an anesthetic antiseptic like Chloraseptic, you can easily get some of the spray on the patient's tongue. Then the patient's throat may feel better, but he has the discomfort of a numb tongue.

To prevent a numb tongue, invert the bowl of a teaspoon over the patient's tongue and then spray his throat. The spoon not only protects his tongue from the spray, but also depresses his tongue so you can see the area of his throat that's red and sore.

—LINDA BARKER, RN

THE POP THAT REFRESHES

Patients on fluid restrictions have thirsts to satisfy, like anyone else. But small quantities of liquids that get swallowed in one sip aren't very satisfying.

To quench patients' thirsts and still keep accurate intake/output records, make "Popsicles" from juice or an allowed supplement. Pour the liquid into 30-ml cups, insert an orange wood stick in each, and then put the cups into a freezer. When you're ready to use the "Popsicles," loosen the cups by running them under warm water for a few seconds. Patients really enjoy these treats, and they stay within their fluid limits.

—MARY MASSARO, RN

TUBE TWIST

Whenever you need to clamp a naso-gastric tube briefly (for instance, to ambulate the patient, between feedings, and so forth), use the tube itself as the clamp. Just fold the tubing 6 inches (15

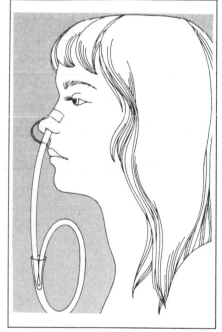

cm) from the end and insert this folded portion into the opening.

This handy maneuver saves time spent looking for clamps and doesn't strain the tubing with the added weight of a normal clamp.

—DEBRA SCHMALTZ, RN, BS

BEDPAN EASE

If using a bedpan is too awkward for your patients in traction, try this.

Put a stadium chair (the kind with only a seat and backrest—no legs) on the patient's bed. Place the bedpan on the chair. The patient can help transfer himself on and off the bedpan by using a trapeze.

The chair supports the patient's back, making the bedpan routine more comfortable and less awkward. (Of course, this method works only for patients who can sit up or bend at the hip.)

—CECELIA MOORE, RN

A HAIR-RAZING LIFT

One grooming practice to enhance a mastectomy patient's self-image is shaving her legs.

Have her use this easy way to get a smooth shave without using soap or shave cream, or having to rinse off with water. First, have her wet her legs with a washcloth. Then apply a thin film of lotion or baby oil and proceed to shave.

This procedure is simple enough for you to do on patients. But the patient shaving her legs herself makes her feel better than having someone else do it for her.

—LINDA S. BATES, RN

SNAG SOLUTION

Many postop patients wear elastic abdominal binders for support in coughing, deep breathing, and ambulating. The binders' Velcro linings are great for adjusting the binders to fit properly, but the lining causes a problem for some women. After surgery, they like to wear their own nylon nightgowns; but the

Velcro catches and snags the material, ruining the gowns.

To solve this problem, cover the exposed Velcro with gauze. Besides eliminating needless wear and tear on the patients' nightgowns, the gauze guides you in reapplying the binder after a dressing change or ambulation. A timesaver for you—no more readjustments for proper fit—and a gownsaver for patients.

—JANET POSPY, RN, BSN

REFRESHING SQUIRT

A patient with second- and third-degree burns on his face has lips so sensitive that he can't put a straw or the rim of a cup against them. He can, though, use a syringe to squirt liquids into his mouth without touching his lips.

Fill several 50-ml sterile syringes with juice, milk, or water and leave them in ice at his bedside. Then, when he wants a drink, he can serve himself—you don't need to return to isolation.

—MELODY L. ZIOBRO, RN

IRRIGATION PROJECT

When patients have advanced oral cancer, their lesions give off foul-smelling secretions. To reduce odors and keep patients clean and comfortable, irrigate their lesions regularly.

A primary concern is to reach every oral cavity. So apply solution from a catheter-tip syringe or a disposable enema bag with tubing, rather than simply rinsing from a cup.

For each irrigation, use at least 1 quart (0.95 liter) of either half-strength hydrogen peroxide and astringent mouthwash, or sodium bicarbonate and warm water in a mild solution, followed by clean tap water. Whichever solution you use, try to irrigate regularly—once every 4 hours that the patient's awake.

These methods work especially well when patients' lesions open to the outside of the face or neck. Then the solution comes through these openings to clean the lesions without damaging surrounding tissue.

—NANCY DELANO, RN

MENDING MATTERS

Here's how to fix the cut or damaged balloon-inflation line (or cuff-inflation line) of an endotracheal tube so the tube doesn't have to be replaced.
1. Pull back the needle of a 20-gauge catheter and cut the catheter at the same angle as the needle. Then slide the needle forward again so its bevel is flush with the cut catheter.
2. Cut off the damaged portion of the line, and insert the catheter into one part of the line. (The submerged needle will guide the catheter, without tearing through the line.) Remove the needle from the catheter and cut the other end of the catheter at an angle. Insert this end into the other part of the line.
3. Tape the connections securely.

Now you've repaired the line without causing the patient unnecessary discomfort or expense.

—RANDY H. FINLEY, RN, BSN

SIP TIP

If you don't have enough hands or help to wrestle with a glass of water *and* a reluctant patient while you insert a nasogastric tube, try this. Have the patient just sip on a straw. This action directs the tube into the esophagus rather than the trachea. That achieves the desired result—with no water going to the N.P.O. patient, and no wet gowns, either.

—MARY JANE CRAIG, RN

ALL STRAPPED IN

Use Montgomery straps to secure Foley catheters. First, cut a 4x4-inch (10x10-cm) section from a Montgomery strap. Then into the section's center, cut two parallel ¼-inch (.63-cm) slits an inch (2.5-cm) apart. After weaving the string supplied with the strap through the slits, apply the strap's sticky side to the patient and tie the string around the catheter.

This simple device can all but eliminate the need to reposition Foley catheters. So you'll save yourself time and your patients considerable discomfort.

—JACQUELINE KASULANIS, RN

A ROUTINE CHANGE

When a Gomco suction machine isn't suctioning well—or at all—don't reposition the patient or his nasogastric tube until you've checked the collection bottle.

If the bottle has more than 1,000 ml of drainage, the machine doesn't work efficiently. So routinely change the bottle when the contents reach this point, and you may not have to disturb the patient.

—KIMBERLY ANTON, LPN

CUE CARDS

If a cardiac arrest is a rare event in your hospital, at the beginning of each shift

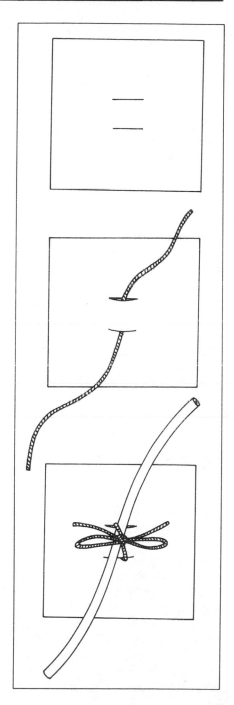

distribute five "Code Blue" cards: cards listing specific duties the cardholder will perform in the event of a cardiac arrest. The five roles include: team leader, ventilator, compressor, medication and recording nurse, and runner.

Now you'll know what your job is *before* an arrest occurs, and you can help the patient more quickly—without losing time because of confusion and missed cues.

—JO AZZARELLO, RN

SPONGING OFF

For patients who have one arm or one hand immobilized, using a washcloth is difficult. A sponge is easier for such patients to handle. It fits right into the hand, can be wrung out easily, and doesn't require folding as a washcloth does. Patients feel more independent, giving their own sponge baths.

A sponge is also effective for arthritic patients, since the squeezing action helps loosen up stiff joints.

—VICKI PRECHENENKO, RN

NO CATH? NO PROBLEM

When you have a male patient who's incontinent of urine, but can't use an indwelling urinary catheter, try a newborn-size disposable diaper instead.

Just gently wrap the diaper around the patient's entire penis, secure the tape tab, and fold over or tape the open end shut.

The disposable diapers are more comfortable and safer than conventional incontinent pants and pins, and they look better under trousers than bulky rubber pants. Also, after the pa-

tient has voided, you can weigh the diaper for an accurate intake and output measurement. And before applying a fresh diaper, all you (or he) need do is clean the genital area.

—JUDITH B. SCHWANDT, RN

CATH PATCH

To patch a cracked hub in a Swan-Ganz catheter, thread a 20-gauge angiocath into the hub's porthole, then remove the angiocath needle. (Don't pierce the Swan-Ganz tubing with the needle.)

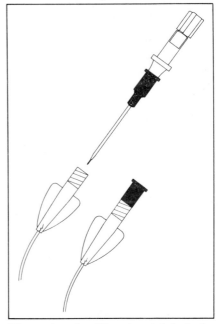

The angiocath will wedge tightly in the porthole and form a seal bypassing the cracked hub.

—DEBRA C. DAVIS, RN, MSN

URINE-FREE CAST

To prevent urine contamination of a hip-spica cast, cover its crotch area with a polyethylene drape. The drape's hypoallergenic adhesive sticks to the cast and won't irritate the patient's skin.

—ANN CUNNINGHAM, RN

BAG IT

The drainage collection devices used after surgery can irritate your patient's skin when they're taped on and changed often. To avoid the discomfort of tape, take a 6-inch (15-cm) piece of stockinette, seal one end to form a bag, and insert the collection device. Then attach the bag to the patient's dressing, or else make a gauze belt to hold the bag in place.

Because the bag stays in place without tape, you can change the collection devices whenever necessary and not worry about hurting your patient.

—LOUISE SWEETEN, RN

SPLINT HINT

Urinary pouches may twist and develop leaks when connected to a gravity drainage device. But a splint—made from a 1x3-inch (2.5x7.5-cm) piece of stiff plastic, cardboard, or tongue blade—can help prevent this.

Just tape the splint across the pouch's lower edge, about 1 inch (2.5 cm) above the outlet. The splint will help maintain the bag's shape, keep it from twisting, and give the ostomate peace of mind knowing his bag won't leak.

—JOYCE DOWNING, RN, ET

CIRCUMCISION WRAP

To make a simple, inexpensive dressing for an adult circumcision, unfold a standard 4x4 gauze pad to 4x8. Then fold lengthwise to 2 inches by 8 inches. Coat one side with petroleum jelly, leaving the ends uncoated. Place the coated side along the suture line on the ventral side of the penis and wrap around, crossing the gauze on the dorsal side and taping the ends to the groin.

The tape supports the weight of the dressing, and the patient can void without soiling it.

—TOM MEGOW, SN

WATERMELON MAGIC

When a patient's treatment includes forcing fluids, do you find *yourself* doing the forcing? Solve the fluid problem (at least in the summer months) by serving watermelon. The fruit is loaded with water, cold, nutritious, and patients love it!

—BARBARA NEALE, RN

EYEWASH

Patients with eye traumas need copious eye irrigations. An easy and efficient way to give them is to attach I.V. tubing (without the needle) to 1 liter of normal saline, then use the tubing to direct the saline into the patient's eye. If necessary, you can regulate the stream by using the flow clamp.

—BARBARA SOSAYA, RN, BSN

THE TIE THAT'S KIND

Obviously, taping a nasal endotracheal tube (ETT) to a burn patient's face is bound to cause additional skin irritation. So instead of taping the ETT on, tie it on as follows:

Cut both ends off a #14 French (or larger) suction catheter. Then cut the catheter into two pieces—each as long as the distance from your patient's nose to his ear.

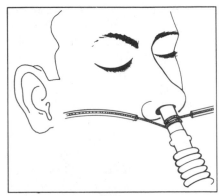

Next, thread umbilical tape (long enough to tie around the patient's head) through both catheter pieces. To simplify threading, use an 18-gauge needle to push the tape through both catheters' lumens.

Wet the outside of the ETT with benzoin to make it sticky. Loop the tape—the part *between* the two catheter pieces—around the ETT. Then secure the ETT by tying the tape ends behind the patient's head.

This kind of tie will stay clean longer than tape. Best of all, it won't rub or pull your patient's delicate skin.

—ADRIANA SULLENGER, RN

FOAM IN THE MOUTH

To remove blood from a patient's mouth, try a solution of half peroxide and half ginger ale. Just dip a toothbrush, mouth swab, or gauze into the solution, brush or wipe the patient's mouth, and let the blood foam away. Follow with a plain water rinse.

This method works especially well on unconscious patients. And most conscious patients find it a pleasant mouth rinse.

—JANICE HEISTAND, RN, CCRN

STRETCH STORAGE

If your recovery room patients need an emesis basin or some tissues—stat, but these items aren't close at hand, ask the maintenance department to make and attach small metal trays under the head of each stretcher. Then store supplies on the trays, and they're always within reach, p.r.n.

—EMILY NICKLES, RN

REMADE MASKS

Many patients refuse to wear their one-size-fits-all oxygen masks because these masks are simply too large and uncomfortable: The plastic rim juts into the patient's eyes and allows air to escape.

To tailor the mask, trim the top edge a bit and cover it with cloth tape. With a comfortable custom-fit mask, the patients become more compliant with their oxygen therapy.

—JERENE MAUNE, RN

GIVE 'EM A BOOT

Give your patients with temporary transvenous pacemakers a boot—a Buck's traction boot, that is.

Simply place the patient's arm and the pulse generator in the boot, and fasten the straps to keep the arm immobile. If the patient's arm is longer than the boot, cut open the end of the boot. And, with confused patients, tie the boot to the bed with the attached traction rope.

The boot's metal strip keeps the arm straight but less rigid than it would be with a conventional armboard. Also, the pulse generator can be kept alongside rather than on top of the arm, adding to patient comfort.

Keep a Buck's traction boot on your pacemaker cart, since it's just the boot some patients need.

—JOAN BELISLE, RN

HEADS UP

Sometimes a stroke patient has trouble holding his head up while sitting, which makes feeding him difficult and limits his view of his surroundings. Here are two solutions to this problem, depending on the patient's needs.

1. Refold a 3x4-inch (7.5x10-cm) folded dressing lengthwise to make it 1½x8 inches (3.8x20 cm), and put it across the patient's forehead like a headband or sweatband. Then, run a piece of 1-inch (2.5-cm) tape across the headband and fasten it to the back of the chair behind the patient's head. While the tape holds the patient's head up, it doesn't touch his skin—and the "headline" supporting him isn't obvious to passersby.

2. Apply a cervical collar, perhaps cut a bit narrower than standard width. The collar especially helps if the patient's mouth droops on one side. With his chin resting on the soft collar, the patient can keep his mouth comfortably shut, lessening drooling.

These supports lift a patient's morale as well as his head.

—ELIZABETH GAVULA, RN

INSIDE POCKET

Ambulating patients with a Hemovac can be a problem. The solution? A secret inside pocket.

Pin a washcloth to the inside of the patient's robe to form a pocket. Then tell the patient to *drop* (not pin) the Hemovac into the pocket when he gets out of bed.

This way, the Hemovac is out of sight and safe from being pulled out.

—LINDA MITCHELL, RN

NICKEL'S WORTH

After eye surgery, a patient may have dressings over both eyes and have trouble finding the nurse's call button on the bedside console. Tape a nickel on top of the button to help the patient identify it. Then he need only run his fingers over the console until he feels the familiar coin, and press the button.

—DARYL SEIFERT, RN

A GOOD SHAKE

When a patient wants—and *needs*—a high-calorie, high-protein bedtime snack, but the hospital's kitchen is closed, what can you do? Take a look at the snacks stored in your unit's refrigerator and improvise.

For example, you can mix a carton or two of any flavor of ice cream with milk for a quick, nutritious, and appetizing milk shake. (Let the ice cream soften slightly first for easier mixing.) Or mix some sherbet with a liquid elemental diet, such as Vivonex. Patients will like these shakes—and benefit from their nutritional value too.

—VICKI EPHROU, RN

NOW HEAR THIS

You've probably heard of—or tried—using a stethoscope to talk to a hard-of-hearing patient. That is, you place the earpieces in the patient's ears and speak clearly, in low tones, into the bell. But here's another way to bridge a communication gap with a stethoscope.

If you're caring for a patient who has a tracheostomy, is receiving mechanical ventilation, or for some other reason can't talk, use the stethoscope this way: Place the bell on the patient's lips and the earpieces in your ears. Then ask the patient to whisper. His words will come in—loud and clear.

—JOANNE BOUSQUET, GN

SKIN LOTION POTION

Cleaning dried fecal material from an incontinent patient is difficult. But a small amount of skin lotion applied with a soft cloth easily removes the material and prevents the dryness that soap can cause—even after rinsing with plain water. This technique is especially good for elderly patients and those with dry or fragile skin.

—ELAINE M. NEIDERT, SN

ONE-STEP TRANSFER

Here's how to weigh and transfer a semicomatose, obese patient to a new bed. Use a bed scale for the weighing. Then, with the patient still on the scale and two more nurses stationed at his head and feet, push the bed out from under the patient and slide the new bed—all made up—underneath in its place. Then move him off the scale and onto the new bed.

The whole procedure takes about 5 minutes and is easy on your back and your patient's delicate skin.

—C. DEBRA STRUTMAN, RN

KITCHEN CREAM

Since diabetics need to take special care of their feet, tell them they probably have an effective, inexpensive cream right in their own kitchen that'll help soften their dry, calloused skin. It's solid vegetable shortening.

Tell the diabetic to put a dab of shortening in the palm of his hand after bathing. Then have him add a few drops of water and mix with the shortening until he gets a nice cream that rubs in well and doesn't leave a greasy covering. Using this treatment once or twice a day will bring dramatic results. What's more, the "cream" can be used on elbows, hands, knees—wherever rough skin is a problem.

—JOYCE A. MCCARTHY, RN

NO-MESS MOUTH CARE

Giving mouth care to a patient who must lie flat in bed isn't easy—especially the rinsing and spitting. But here's a way to avoid the mess.

After the patient's teeth are brushed, offer him mouthwash or water through a straw. Then, have him use the same straw to expel the mouthwash or water into an emesis basin.

Although using a straw may be a bit awkward at first, patients usually master it quickly and become proficient in the ins *and* outs of rinsing and spitting with straws.

—KATHY SCHEEVE, SN

DRAINING DRY

Ever care for a patient who'd had a ventricular drainage catheter removed? The catheter site on his forehead continues to drain cerebrospinal fluid, requiring dressing changes every 1 to 2 hours.

So improvise a drainage system. Put

a sterile, disposable pediatric urine collector over the catheter site and connect the collector's drainage tube to an empty, sterile I.V. bag.

This device not only eliminates a possible source of infection—the wet dressings—but it also serves as a sterile, closed drainage system to measure the cerebrospinal fluid.

—VIVIAN E. LYONS, RN

FILL IN THE BLANKS

If you have a patient who's paralyzed or immobilized and must spend a lot of time in a side-lying position to prevent decubiti, here's a way to help him. Make an inexpensive magazine or book holder to attach to the bed so the patient can read rather than just stare at the wall. The holder is ideal for one-page articles, poems, or letters.

First, get one of those report cover kits with clear plastic sheets and plastic slide locks. (They're available at most variety stores or drugstores.) Cut two of the plastic sheets about 3 inches (7.5 cm) longer and 1 inch (2.5 cm) wider than the book or magazine that will go into the holder. Next, staple the sheets together on three sides to make an envelope or pouch.

Then, cut the slide locks to fit the envelope's sides and bottom (miter the adjoining edges of the slide locks for a tighter fit). With a hot ice pick or small drill, make two holes in each slide lock. Lace a 4-ply yarn through the holes, leaving about 8 inches (20 cm) on each side and on the bottom to loop around the top and bottom bed rails.

Finally, tie the holder to the bed rails, adjust it to the patient's eye level, and slip in the book or magazine. The holder won't hamper the bed rails' movement. Best of all, because the materials just slide in, you can vary the

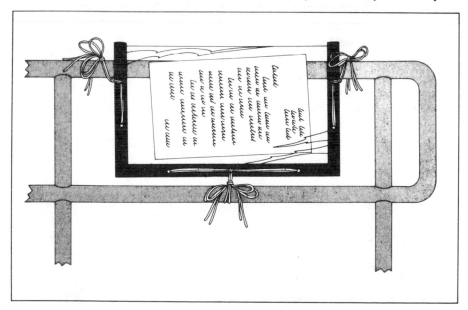

patient's "side-show"—and keep boredom at bay—with just a flip of your wrist.

—Pat Baggerly, RN

VENTILATION PREPARATION

Picture this: A patient with a laryngectomy is admitted to the ICU. You soon learn that he hasn't worn his laryngectomy tube for years, and the respiratory therapists can't insert a tube. So you worry that if the patient has a cardiac arrest, you'd have only one way to ventilate him—mouth to stoma resuscitation. You couldn't place him on the ventilator or deliver any high oxygen concentration to him.

The solution? Place an endotracheal tube into his stoma just far enough to get a seal. This will allow you to ventilate him with a manual resuscitation bag or place him on a mechanical ventilator.

—Marti Brown, RN

COLORFUL SIGNALS

When a patient with a tracheostomy takes fluids orally for the first time, do you worry about aspiration? Deciding which secretions he's coughing up—tracheobronchial or clear fluids in danger of being aspirated—isn't easy.

So, give colorful fluids, such as red gelatin or grape juice, instead of clear fluids. These colorful signals help identify the secretions and protect the patient.

—Michael Couillard, RN

CUT FOR COMFORT

For patients who've had radical neck surgery, hospital gowns just won't do.

They're too tight around the patient's neck, causing pressure on suture lines and Hemovac sites, and they cover the tracheostomy opening, obstructing the patient's airway.

Unsnapping or untying the top fastener helps—but the gown may then fall off the patient's shoulders.

So make a slight alteration—cut a 4x4-inch (10x10-cm) section out of the front of the neckband—and rehem the band. These altered hospital gowns serve patients well.

—Rita Sauer, RN

A FOLEY FIX

If a patient with a Foley catheter complains that his leg drainage bag bunches up, make two simple alterations. First,

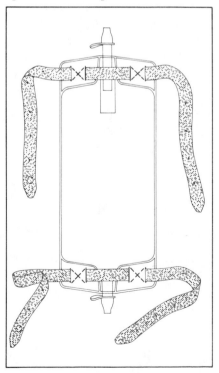

cut four extra slits—two at the top of the bag and two at the bottom, each about an inch (2.5 cm) from one of the existing slits.

Next, thread the bag's top strap through the top four slits and sew the strap to the bag at the two threading points. Thread and sew the bottom strap the same way. Now, the bag stays securely attached to the strap and doesn't ride up.

Note: When passing this tip on to your patients, warn them to be careful not to puncture the drainage pouch when slitting the bag.

—JEANNE SULLIVAN, RN

BELOW AND BAGGED

Patients on constant urinary drainage have a double problem when ambulating: First, they forget the importance of keeping the drainage bag at a level below the bladder. Second, they're embarrassed by the appearance of the bag itself.

To avoid these problems, take an attractive opaque plastic bag with a drawstring closure, and place the urinary drainage container in this bag. The opaque bag is just the right length when held by its string to keep the urinary container below the bladder, and the bag keeps the patient from being embarrassed.

—NOREEN E. BREACH, RN

EASY-OFF TAPE

To secure an endotracheal tube without getting tape stuck in your patient's hair, do this:

Cut a piece of 1-inch (2.5-cm) tape about 24 inches (60 cm) long. Cut an-

other piece about 9 inches (22.5 cm) long. With the sticky sides facing each other, center the shorter piece over the longer piece and press the pieces together.

Now place the tape under the patient's head (double-thick section at the back of his head) and bring the ends around the tube, securing it in place.

This technique holds the tube in place, and you won't pull the patient's hair when you take the tape off.

—BETTY HORVATH, RN

BRING ON THE BRAN

No one—neither patient nor nurse—enjoys a laxative or an enema. Yet, for long-term bedridden patients on a solid food diet, establishing bowel habits presents problems.

Here's a solution to some of those problems—unprocessed bran. With patients who are immobile for long periods and who have no dietary restrictions, sprinkle 1 to 2 teaspoons of bran on their food or in their fruit juice for each meal daily. Then leave the bran container at their bedside so they can regulate the amount to suit their own needs, perhaps decreasing it to twice daily. Patients using bran have no cramping, as they do after a laxative, and they don't have discomfort. And, oh, the nursing hours saved by the decreased need for enemas!

—MYRA B. ALEXANDER, RN

TUBE TRICK

If you have patients who must be tube fed through a small jejunostomy tube, here's a way to set up a continuous system that's also nearly leakproof. Remove the rubber top from a sterile eye dropper and discard the top. Insert the dropper end into the jejunostomy tube. Then connect a piece of suction tubing (about 4 inches [10 cm] long) to the neck of the eye dropper. Connect the other end of the suction tubing to the adapter of the tube feeding setup, and the system is ready to go.

—WANDA TULLIER, SN

SNIP 'N SHRIVEL

For the patient with a Sengstaken-Blakemore tube in place, the possibility of the esophageal balloon's slipping upward, causing the patient to suffocate, poses a threat. As a safeguard, keep a pair of scissors taped to the head of the bed for emergencies. If immediate deflation becomes necessary, cut the inflation tube and release the pressure. Although this happens rarely, life hangs in the balance, so be prepared.

—BRIGID JAYNES, RN

ATTENTION-GETTER

Tape a square of washed X-ray film to the front of patients' charts to make a see-through pocket for messages or reminders to the doctor. Cut a large notch in the open end so notes can be inserted

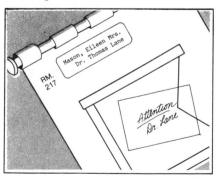

and removed easily. The pockets also serve as holders for identification plates of patients who are sent to surgery.

—DIANE KLAIBER, RN

EMERGENCY TAPES

Before a patient with a laryngectomy is discharged, pass on this helpful—sometimes lifesaving—hint: Ask a relative or friend to tape-record several "emergency" phone messages that can be played over the phone to the fire company, police department, ambulance service, or doctor.

The messages might say: "My name is *(patient's name)*, I live at *(his address)*. I'm a laryngectomy patient and need a *(doctor's, ambulance's, or whatever)* assistance at *(repeat address)*. Please notify *(name of friend or relative)* at *(phone number)*."

Tell patients to mark all tapes clearly (only one message should be recorded on each side of a tape) and to keep the tapes and emergency phone numbers by their phones.

The messages allow patients who live alone or are alone for long periods of time to be independent and confident that they can get help if needed.

—SUZANNE S. STEPHENS, RN

LACERATION LUBRICATION

If a scalp laceration is hard to suture because the patient's hair gets entangled in the suture material (even though the wound area has been prepped), try this technique. After you've shaved the area, apply Lubafax, or a similar sterile, water-soluble lubricant, around the hairline of the laceration. This will hold the hair down, preventing it from getting entangled in the suture and providing a more sterile field. The lubricant can be easily washed out after suturing.

—LINDA DRAIN, RN
CHERYL WESTBAY, RN

PLASTIC-WRAP PATTERN

Before applying an ostomy pouch to a large draining wound, you may have to enlarge the opening in the adhesive backing. Here's a quick, accurate way to measure the wound and to cut an opening that'll fit around the wound without touching it.

Place a piece of plastic wrap over the wound. On the plastic, outline the wound with a broad, felt-tip marking pen. Mark the patient's top, left, and right sides.

Next, cut out the plastic-wrap pattern and place it with the marked side down over the opening in the pouch's backing. This way you don't reverse the pattern. Center the pattern as much as possible over the opening.

Trace the pattern on the paper covering the backing. Then cut the pattern out of paper *and* backing, and remove this section. Now, when you affix the backing to the patient's skin, the opening will accurately fit around the wound.

—LYNDA L. BRUBACHER, RN, ET

A HINT OF MINT

Here's how to absorb strong odors caused by a patient's draining wound or profuse bleeding.

Take three or four cotton balls and put a few drops of peppermint oil on each ball. Then put the balls in a plastic medicine cup and place the cup in the patient's room, usually on a windowsill.

Change the balls every day, so the peppermint oil keeps the patient's room smelling fresh.

—SISTER FREDERICA, RN

PATENT IDEA

Copious gastrointestinal bleeding may clog a nasogastric tube despite hourly irrigations. To keep the tube patent, use this technique on the half hour.

Sandwich the tube between two tongue blades, placed lengthwise about 15 inches

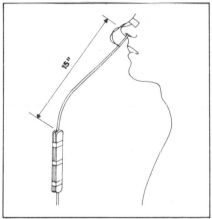

(37.5 cm) from the nares. Fasten the blades with silk tape—just tight enough to keep them in place. Then, press the blades together to dislodge clots.

—JOY MURRAY, RN

SEALED FOR SAFETY

Do you keep a crash cart between medical units, where it's easily accessible? And during routine equipment checks, do you occasionally find that someone borrowed an item and forgot to replace it?

With the help of the maintenance department, insert heavy-duty staples into the frame of the cart, below each of the drawers. Then wrap 10-inch (25-cm) wire around the staples and the drawer handles to seal the drawers shut.

The wires break with very little exertion, so the drawers are still easy to open. But now you know at a glance whether they've been opened and if crucial supplies might be missing.

—NANCY BONNE, RN

AVOIDING PROBLEMS

If you care for incontinent male patients—some comatose, others paralyzed from the waist down—here's how to keep both bed and patient dry without risking urinary tract infection from catheterization.

Cut a 2-inch (5-cm) slot in a bed liner and place it (absorbent side down) over the patient's pubis. Slip the patient's penis through the slot and position a urinal. If urine dribbles or the urinal overflows onto the polyethylene side, the urine won't soak through to the patient or the bed.

—RALPH VOGEL, RN

OUCHLESS TAPING

Here's how to keep Montgomery straps in place without taping the straps to the patient's skin. Cut a piece of Stomahesive, a little larger than the tape, and apply the adhesive side to the patient's skin (preferably, to a flat surface). Then tape the Montgomery straps to the Stomahesive.

Using this method, you can remove the tape from the shiny side of the Stomahesive several times to change dressings without traumatizing the patient's skin.

—LYNDA BRUBACHER, RN, ET

DRY DRESSING

If your patient has constant leakage around the cystostomy tubes, use half of a toddler-sized disposable diaper as a dressing. The diaper's liner draws wetness away from the patient's skin, and its outer layer of plastic protects his clothing. Put extra padding inside the dressing if needed. Tape around the edges keeps the dressing in place for 2 days.

—JOANN TERVENSKI, RN, BS

UP AND AWAY

A patient with diabetic gangrene may complain of discomfort from the pressure of the covers about his foot. If a foot cradle isn't available, lay a light-

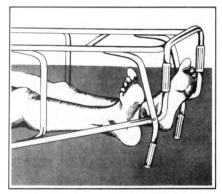

weight aluminum walker on the bed to support the covers.

—PEGGY KREIZINGER
SHIRLEY A. BRINSON, RN

JELLY REMOVER

Removing dried electrode jelly from a patient's skin can be difficult—especially if the patient has sensitive skin. Instead of using acetone, which is abrasive, use A and D Ointment.

Apply the ointment generously, and

leave it on the skin for a few minutes before rubbing it in. With babies, apply the ointment before bathing them and remove it after their bath. Besides removing the jelly, the ointment also helps heal the skin.

—LINDA MILEWSKI, RN, BSN

BILINGUAL POSTER

If no one on the staff can communicate with foreign-speaking patients, try a visual approach to the problem—a bilingual poster.

Choose a few important words, like bath, pain, food, and water, and write them in both the foreign language and English. Then hang the posters in patients' rooms, in plain sight.

The posters not only help break down the communication barrier, but also give both patients and staff a good laugh whenever someone mispronounces a word.

—PAM BARTON, RN

HEAD SUPPORT

Here's a way to provide head support for debilitated patients so they can sit in an armchair or wheelchair.

First, position the patient comfortably and safely, with his body in proper alignment. Next, wrap a 2- to 3-inch (5- to 7.5-cm) felt collar twice around his neck. Then, apply a well-padded cotton halter under the patient's chin, padding the sides of the halter with cotton strips or bandages, to protect the patient's face. Attach the other ends of the cotton strips or bandages to an I.V. pole placed behind the patient. Using this method, the patient can still swivel his head to see what's going on around him.

This technique strengthens the neck muscles and boosts the patient's morale as well as his head.

—LUCY DALICANDRO, RN

OSTOMY AID

Patients with reusable ostomy equipment may have trouble removing the double-face adhesive disk from the faceplate when they want to clean their appliances. Here's a tip to make removal easier:

Tell the patient to apply Skin Prep protective dressing (the brush-on, spray-on, or wipe-on kind) to the faceplate and allow the dressing to dry for 1 or 2 minutes. Make sure the faceplate is covered evenly. (If he's using the spray, tell him to spread the dressing with his finger after spraying.) The patient can then apply the adhesive disk to the faceplate and proceed as usual.

The Skin Prep gives the faceplate a clean coating that makes the disk easy to remove. It helps to keep faceplates in good condition longer, too.

—PATRICIA A. NIGRO, RN, ET

DRAINAGE BAG DILEMMA

Placing a urinary drainage bag in the correct position when a patient is in a wheelchair can be difficult. Either the bag is hung so high it's above the patient's bladder, or so low it's dragging on the floor.

Solve this problem by inserting a grommet (a metal eyelet) through the vinyl backing of the wheelchair—at the center bottom of the chair back—and placing a small "S" hook through the hole in the grommet. Then hang the drainage bag from the hook. This method keeps the bag below the patient's bladder, but away from the floor.

—DIANNE E. DUNNE, RN

TENT THE TUBE

Drainage that leaks out *around* abdominal sump or gastrostomy tubes causes wet bedclothes and skin irritation.

To prevent this, use a "tented" tube-and-pouch device, which calls for the following procedures:

Obtain a skin barrier (such as Karaya or Stomahesive), a drainable ostomy pouch with an adhesive backing, and reinforcing tape. In the centers of the

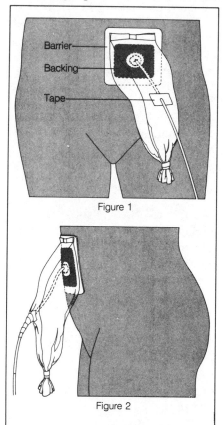

Barrier
Backing
Tape

Figure 1

Figure 2

barrier and the pouch adhesive, cut openings no more than ¼ inch (.6 cm) larger than the opening in the patient's abdomen.

Now turn the pouch around. Place a piece of tape about 1 inch (2.5 cm) lower than the bottom edge of the adhesive on the pouch's other side. Then cut a hole, slightly smaller than the tube diameter, through the tape and pouch.

To apply the barrier, first clean and dry the patient's skin. Then disconnect the suction momentarily, slip the barrier over the tube, and affix the barrier to the patient.

Next, thread the tube through the hole in the pouch adhesive, then out through the tape-reinforced hole on the pouch's other side. Affix the pouch back securely to the skin barrier.

Now return to the pouch front and wrap tape around the tube where it passes through the tape-reinforced hole. Be sure the tape covers the area *between* the tube and pouch hole where drainage could leak. Continue to wrap tape about 4 inches (10 cm) up the tube. Fasten the end of the pouch as you would with any drain.

Besides sealing the tube opening, this "tented" tube-in-pouch device serves as a splint to reduce tension on the tube. It also allows you to empty and rinse the pouch from the end, without disturbing the taped seal between tube and pouch. As a result, your patient stays drier, cleaner, and more comfortable.

—CARLEEN D. PARLATO, RN, ET

A WAY WITH WOUNDS

Paint deep abrasions with lidocaine (lignocaine, Xylocaine) to relieve pain before you scrub or suture them. (Of course, first get a doctor's order to use this drug.) Then use a surgical scrub brush to remove all dirt particles from the wound. Finally, to help the patient keep his wound clean at home, pack a few disposable soap pads in a take-along bag.

—BONITA L. MITCHELL, RN

EASY AND ASEPTIC

After suctioning with a disposable suction catheter, wrap the catheter around your gloved hand, disconnect it from the connecting tube and take the glove off, making sure that the catheter remains inside the little bag formed by the glove. This is an easy and aseptic way to dispose of used suction catheters.

—GAIL FINE

HIGHTOPS

Footdrop in comatose, paralyzed, or bedridden patients can be prevented by using footboards, but working with them is awkward and cumbersome. After trying a number of preventive methods, high-topped canvas basketball sneakers seem to work best.

First put a pair of socks on the patient, then snugly lace up the sneakers. To keep the feet aired and dry, keep the sneakers on 4 hours, then off 4 hours.

It's also much easier to turn and position the patient wearing sneakers rather than work with boards and bolsters.

—CAROL SCHREIBER, RN

BEDPAN LINING

When careful stool measurements are ordered for a patient with gross rectal bleeding, try collecting specimens this way. First, rinse a bedpan with water. Next, press a large plastic bag into the contours of the pan, so the bag's edges form a collar over the edge of the pan. (The moisture in the pan keeps the bag in place.)

After the patient has passed the stool, lift the bag out of the pan and place it in the measuring container. Neither blood nor stool clings to either the bedpan or the container. This increases accuracy while eliminating cleanup.

To reduce odor, twist and tie the bag. You can save the specimen in a tied bag without telltale odors or much change in color.

—RUTH P. WHITNEY, RN

CANE KEEPER

Since many nursing home residents use canes, geriatric nurses spend precious time retrieving canes that fall to the floor or behind a piece of furniture. Use pinch-mop holders to keep the canes from slipping away. Have the maintenance department attach a holder to each resident's bedside stand. These holders work especially well on canes that don't have hooked handles, and they keep all canes within easy reach of residents and staff.

—PAT GAMMEL, RN

LEG HOLDER

When you change dressings on a patient with leg burns, you need another person to hold the patient's leg—until you use this system. Ask the maintenance department to make a leg holder. Have them solder a piece of pipe to the frame of a metal foot cradle, then anchor the pipe under the mattress. Now, one person can elevate the patient's leg, place it in the holder, and inspect and change the dressings. What's more, the holder's comfortable for patients, too.

—KATHY GEORGE, RN

ENEMA TACTICS

Have a problem using disposable enemas for elderly patients because of lax rectal sphincters or large hemorrhoids? To get the fluid well into the rectum, slide an ordinary rectal tube onto the tip of the disposable container before using it.

—E. ROGERS

GET THE PICTURE?

Here's an aid to repositioning paraplegic and brain-injured patients without having to ask for assistance. Use printed diagrams showing a body in various positions to indicate where padding should go. After the admitting nurse checks the patient's bone structure and examines him for paralysis and decu-

biti, she draws arrows on the diagram to show pressure points that should be padded. She also briefly describes what kind of padding is needed (*small pad, large pillow,* and so forth). Then, referring to the diagram, an aide can safely and comfortably reposition patients without the nurse's help.

—JEAN SORRELL, RN

TAKING THE GUESSWORK OUT OF ESTIMATING BLEEDING

When you phone a doctor to report a patient's bleeding, do you have trouble describing how much? Many nurses do. Estimating isn't easy. Terms such as "bleeding heavily" could mean anywhere from 10 ml per hour to five or ten times that much.

To avoid this problem, use a visual aid.

Take three perineal pads. Onto the first, place 10 ml of blood from a syringe; onto the second, 30 ml; and onto the third, 60 ml. Then lay the three

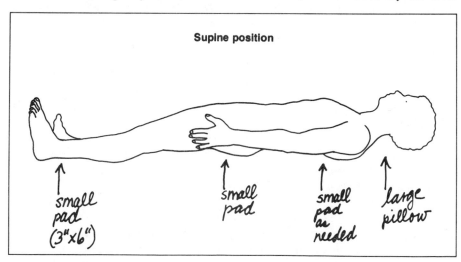

Supine position

small pad (3"x6")   small pad   small pad as needed   large pillow

pads side by side, with cards underneath telling the amounts. Take a color photograph. Enlarge it to 8x10 inches, and place copies on each unit as a ready reference.

—HELEN GRACEY, RN
MICHAEL BRUSER, MD, CRCS(C)

NEUROVASCULAR CHECK CHART

Orthopedic nurses have to check neurovascular signs on postoperative and postcast-application patients every 2, 3, or 4 hours; yet nurses' notes provide space for recording them only once.

To resolve the dilemma, devise a neurovascular checklist on a data sheet, which you'll keep at each patient's bedside. The sheet lists the patient's name, room number, and the orders for checking neurovascular signs—e.g., right leg, q2h x 48 hr. Then list the signs (sensation, temperature, motion, color, edema) in chart form with blanks to be filled in every 2 hours or according to orders. This checklist becomes part of the patient's permanent chart. Although you could use your nurses' notes in this way, the separate chart is easier and allows a more accurate assessment of the patient's neurovascular status.

—LAVERNE M. HAMILL, RN

SKID-PROOF SHOES

For the stroke patient who is just becoming ambulatory, firm, laced shoes with crepe or rubber soles are recommended. But if the patient doesn't have such shoes, you can make his own leather-soled tie shoes skid-proof. Just fit a pair of foam rubber hospital slippers over the patient's shoes and anchor

them with adhesive tape. This will provide both the support and the friction the patient needs to keep from slipping or sliding.

—RENEE BERKE, RN

TAPING TIP

Here's a way to lessen discomfort to patients when you must remove tape from their skin to change dressings, stabilize tubes, and so forth.

When you first apply the tape, fold over one end (sticky sides together) to make a tab. Then when it comes time to remove the tape, you can grasp the starter tab. No need to pick at the tape (and the patient's skin) to get the strip started. You can save still more time and frustration if you leave a tab on the end of the roll of tape for quick access the next time you need it.

—DIANE MAHONEY, RN

BATH-TIME BOLSTER

Pour some baby lotion into the water before bathing a patient. This eliminates the need to apply lotion after washing and drying (which patients appreciate if they're on complete bed rest). Also, baby lotion is an inexpensive substitute for bath oil. Diaphoretic patients especially will appreciate this.

—CHRISTY K. GRECO, LPN

IMPROVISED FOOT CRADLE

If ever you need a foot cradle and find that they've all "disappeared,"... improvise.

Get a cardboard carton from the hospital stockroom and remove the top. If you want to protect the feet, simply cut an opening on one side of the box and place the box over the feet. If you want to protect another part of the body, cut openings on two facing sides and place the box over the area where protection is needed.

Such improvisation is especially helpful for invalids in the home who cannot afford to rent or buy costly equipment.

—NANCY M. CROMBIE, LPN

LENS LIFTER

Ever have to remove contact lenses from multiple trauma patients? The quickest and most painless way to do this is to use the suction tip of a glass eyedropper. By depressing the suction tip and gently applying it directly over the lens, you can lift the lens off the cornea quite easily.

—MARLEEN KAECHELE, RN

PREOP CONSULTATION = POSTOP COOPERATION

Have you ever had a newly postop patient (or his family) oppose you when you tried to carry out your orders for his deep breathing, coughing, or specific exercises?

To avoid this problem, during the visiting hours of the evening preceding surgery, sit with the patient and his family and explain what they might expect *after* the surgery. Mention the possibility of having I.V. fluids, a Foley catheter, nasal oxygen, and try to describe what it will be like to awaken in the recovery room. Tell them the reasons for doing the exercises and for the various equipment that might be used. Answer any questions.

This technique means less apprehen-

sive and more cooperative patients and families after the surgery.

—MARY ANN FOSKO, RN

PUPIL PAPER

Determining a patient's pupil size is an important part of neurologic checks. But in recording the size, terminology may not be specific. For instance, a pupil that appears "moderate" in size to one person, may appear "dilated" to someone else.

To estimate and record pupil size more accurately, make a chart of pupil

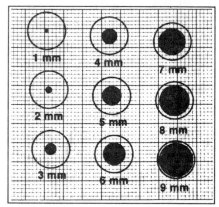

sizes on EKG paper. A pinpoint pupil is 1 mm—the size of one small square. A moderately sized pupil is 5 mm—the size of a large square. A fully dilated pupil is 8 or 9 mm. Keep the pupil-size chart at the nurses' station for quick reference.

—FRANCES MARSHALL, RN

TRACTION PROTECTION

Bars protruding from a traction setup are not only a nuisance, but also dangerous to staff and visitors. Make them injury-proof by placing soft sponge rubber balls on the protruding ends. The balls cushion any contact with the sharp ends. And, since you use bright red balls, people see them from a distance *before* coming in contact with the bars.

—DELLA ANDERSON, RN

CATH CARE COMFORT

Here's a tip for catheterizing a female patient who has a fractured hip or who finds the dorsal recumbent position uncomfortable.

Turn the patient on her left side in the Sims's position, with right knee and thigh drawn up, if possible. Place a sterile drape over her buttocks, covering the rectal area. Then separate the labia and proceed to catheterize her.

Elderly patients especially find this position more comfortable than the traditional position.

—SONJA FEIST, RN, MS

PRACTICE PAD

Teaching a newly diagnosed diabetic to fill a syringe is usually easy. But teaching him to inject the insulin is another story—jabbing the needle into the skin is scary. So, to help patients learn this technique, use an injection practice pad.

Place a foam rubber sponge, measuring 6x8x1½ inches (15x20x3.8 cm), between two sheets of clear plastic about 1 inch (2.5 cm) larger than the sponge. Seal the edges of the plastic with tape. Then, punch holes in the reinforced edges on each end and insert strings for ties. Finally, cut a large target hole in the plastic on one side. Then tie the pad snugly around the patient's upper thigh.

Using ½ ml of sterile water instead

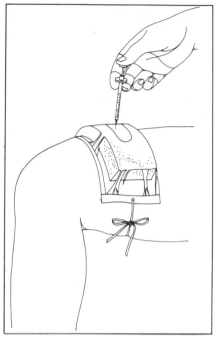

of insulin, the patient can practice injecting the needle through the sponge until he learns the proper direction and force. Placing the pad on his thigh also lets him practice at an actual injection site.

Make these pads in adults' and children's sizes and include one in each teaching kit supplied for diabetics by the central service department.

—MARJORIE B. SHALJEAN, RN

CANE CATCHER

Crutches and canes can fall easily and are difficult to retrieve. For example, if you let go of a cane momentarily to try to prop it somewhere while you're sitting, it's sure to fall to the ground.

Solve this problem by buying a leather dog leash and cutting it down to just a few inches. Then have a shoe repairman stitch the shortened leash around the top of the cane and nail it in place. Slip the patient's arm through the collar, using it just as he'd use a wristlet on a ski pole.

—AGNES MOHNAR, RN

CENT-SAVING SCENT

Have you ever wished you had an effective, pleasant, continuous room deodorizer—for example, when you're caring for new ostomy patients or cancer patients? For such situations, mechanical deodorizing sprays can be overpowering at first and then dissipate quickly. Time-released sprays are expensive.

Oil of cloves can be used as a pleasant, effective, long-lasting deodorizer. Here's how: Pour a small amount of oil of cloves into a glass test tube (the solution eats through plastic). Then dip a 1-inch wide (2.5-cm) gauze wick into the solution and pull one end out over the rim of the test tube.

For the best effect, prepare two such test tubes. Tape one to the foot of the patient's bed and the other to the bathroom wall.

You may also use oil of wintergreen, but it's not as long-lasting and its fragrance is harsher than oil of cloves.

—4 WEST NURSING STAFF
UNIVERSITY OF COLORADO
MEDICAL CENTER

MOBILIZE THE MUSCLES

When you're teaching muscle-toning exercises to orthopedic patients, first demonstrate the exercise on the unaffected side. Then encourage the patient to do the exercises bilaterally. This practice not only retains muscle tone on the uninjured side, but also provides a painless model for the injured side to imitate.

If the patient is timid about moving the injured part, assure him that the doctor has immobilized everything that should not move. Further, what *can* move *should* be exercised so the patient will spend less time in physical therapy regaining use of his muscles once his splint, cast, or traction is removed.

—ADELAIDE H. TATTO, RN

WATCH THE WEIGHT

Are you ever asked to keep accurate records of sputum output for patients who require postural drainage with percussion? If so, you know that transferring a sputum specimen into a graduated cylinder not only gives you inaccurate measurements but also is aesthetically unpleasant.

Weighing rather than measuring specimens is more accurate, more convenient, and more aesthetically pleasing. Use previously weighed plastic drinking cups with lids to collect the specimens. Then, with specimen inside, again weigh the cup on a gram scale. Determine the weight of the sputum by figuring the difference between the two weighings.

Cups with the same lot number are consistent in weight.

—D. JOAN TRAPANI, RN

INNER VIEW

Since many urology patients are unfamiliar with the anatomy of their kidneys and urinary tract, you may have trouble explaining their problem and treatment to them. To help teach them, have some anatomical diagrams printed.

Give each new patient a diagram, explain it and his problem, label the diagram, and leave it with him. The

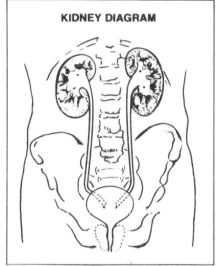

KIDNEY DIAGRAM

patient can review it at his leisure and use it to explain his problem to his family.

If an intravenous pyelogram (I.V.P.) shows a urinary calculus, show its location on the diagram and explain where it will go from there. Also, if subsequent I.V.P.s show the stone's progression, plot its movement on the diagram.

—LINDA MCCLARY, RN

IN THE BAG

If you have a patient with an enema retention problem, position him on his left side at the edge of the bed. (Make sure the side rail is up; you can work through the bars.) Tape an extra-strength plastic bag to the left side of the mattress. Position the patient's buttocks so they rest on the bag's open end,

and place the bottom of the bag in a wastebasket.

Run the enema slowly, allowing waste to drain into the bag. After a short time, turn the patient onto his back to use a bedpan.

This simple method of giving an enema means less mess for you and more comfort for your patient.

—R. E. JACOBSON, RN

STRAW STRETCHER

Drinking without spilling isn't easy for a patient who must lie on his abdomen—even when he's using a straw. To help him, make a "straw stretcher."

Slide the tubing adapter of a 24-inch (60-cm) length of I.V. tubing into the long straight end of a curved drinking straw. Put the I.V. tubing into the patient's glass and let him sip through the curved end of his straw. The tubing extension makes the straw long enough so the patient can drink without tipping his glass and spilling the contents on his bed.

—JEAN SELLERS, RN

CONVERSATION CARDS

If you have patients with communication problems, such as aphasia or a tracheostomy, here's a way to help them. Write messages, such as "I am thirsty," "Please raise my bed," and "I want a drink of water," on index cards. Then punch holes in the cards and attach them to a large key ring so they'll be easy to locate. Patients can quickly communicate their needs or wishes by simply showing you the appropriate card.

You could make several sets of these cards for specific times. For example,

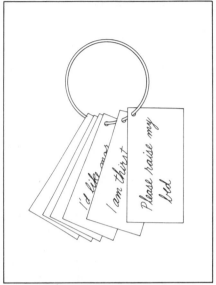

mealtime cards might include such messages as: "I'd like more coffee" and "Please butter my bread." Cards for visiting hours might say: "How is Sandra?" "Is there any mail?" "Who sent the flowers?" You can make other cards that meet a particular patient's needs.

These conversation cards can reduce frustration for both you and your patients.

—KATHLEEN CRUZIE, RN

A CLING THING

Flotation mattresses are beneficial to the patients lying on them, but they can be a real nuisance to the nurses trying to keep the mattresses from slipping off the bed.

To avoid slippage, place a rubber mattress cover over the regular mattress with the reverse (rubber) side up. The plastic covering on the flotation mattress clings to the rubber, so the mattress stays in place. What's more, the patient is more comfortable, and the bed is easier to make.

—KATHY JENNISON, LPN

A THIGH OF RELIEF

If your patient has a leg brace that rubs against the inner thigh of his other leg, avoid this irritation and possible skin breakdown by making a cushion for the normal thigh. Here's how:

Cut off one leg of an old pair of panty hose at midcalf and midthigh to give an open-ended nylon cylinder. Then sew a piece of furlike material (any soft fabric will do) on the cylinder's inner-thigh area.

Now your patient has a padded cylinder that slips on and off his leg easily, doesn't impair circulation, and best of all, protects his skin.

—ETTA M. ROSENTHAL, RN, BS, PHN

STOCKING UP ON EXERCISE

After a mastectomy, the patient is usually instructed to exercise her arm and chest muscles by raising and lowering her arms. An easy way to do this is to put an old nylon stocking over the shower curtain rod, hold the two ends, and pull it in a seesaw motion.

Since the stocking doesn't hurt the rod or the patient's hands, it's a good motivator for *daily* exercise.

—HOLLY M. ROOK, RN

TAGGED BAG

Sometimes when Foley catheter bags are emptied, parts of a 24-hour urine specimen are accidentally thrown out.

To prevent this, place a 1½- to 2-inch (3.8- to 5-cm) piece of adhesive tape across the top of the Foley bag.

Then, using a black felt-tip pen, label the tape with the date and time collection of the 24-hour specimen starts, and the date and time collection is to be completed.

When the test is over, you can remove the tape.

The tape label is small and won't cover the Foley bag's contents, yet it's a constant reminder that urine in the bag should be stored—not thrown out.

—MARY ANN McEVOY, BSN

UNDERCOVER TABLE

Even lightweight bedcovers can rest uncomfortably on the feet of patients who've had orthopedic surgery. To beat this problem after they're discharged from the hospital, tell them to try this:

Put a small, open-legged television table under the top covers, with the tabletop facing the foot of the bed. This keeps the covers off the patient's feet, while allowing enough room for a pillow to elevate the feet. Also, the table-

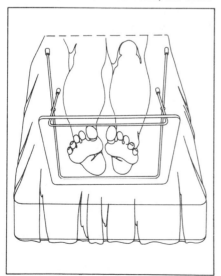

top bottom makes an excellent footrest.

(If the patient doesn't have a table, an empty cardboard box works just as nicely.)

—LYNNE DAVIES, RN

BRIEFLY SPEAKING

To make an inexpensive leg-lift or arm-lift exerciser, sew together the waistband of a man's cotton briefs. Then slip a 5-pound (2.2-kg) bag of sugar (or whatever weight the doctor orders) into the briefs through one leg hole. (Instead of a bag of sugar, you can also use a plastic bag filled with rice or flour.)

Have the patient put his leg through one leg hole of the weighted brief and out the other. Then have him balance the weight on his ankle (or wrist) and begin lifting it up and down. The brief's soft cotton will protect his skin and he can change the weight as his exercise program progresses.

—MARGE KEMPF, RN

DIMINUTIVE DRESSING

Here's a suggestion for postop patients who need just a small dressing or protective cover for their incision when they're discharged. Apply a sanitary pad with an adhesive strip to the undergarment covering the incision. The pad protects the incision, is more economical than a sterile dressing, and has no adhesive touching the skin to irritate the sensitive surgical site (the adhesive strip is attached to the garment).

—CAROL I. LEWIS, RN

VACUUM POWER IN THE E.D.

Use a small, battery-powered vacuum cleaner to remove tiny glass particles from auto accident victims' hair and clothing. The vacuum is more effective than combs and brushes. As an added bonus, it keeps the glass from falling on the floor.

—RICHARD P. KIRSCHKE, RN

NO FALLOUT HERE

Bulky dressings on large or draining abdominal wounds sometimes slip off when patients get out of bed. To avoid this problem, apply Montgomery straps in the conventional manner, i.e., two straps affixed vertically along the wound. Then place a third, smaller, Montgomery strap horizontally below the other straps and lace it through the vertical straps' lower holes. The horizontal strap keeps the dressings in place so the patient can move about confidently.

—CONSTANCE J. GRAMZOW, RN, BSN

CONVERSION CHART

Patients who come to the emergency department may have unwittingly bought centigrade thermometers for home use, but may be unfamiliar with centigrade values. So make a centigrade-Fahrenheit conversion chart, complete with the conversion formula, on a 3x5 card. Send a copy of the chart home with the patients.

Besides saving them the expense of buying a new Fahrenheit thermometer, the chart helps patients get acquainted with the metric system.

—T. HALLINAN, RN

CHECK THE CHART

Do you ever find that another nurse describes a wound drainage as moderate, when you'd consider it small? Or do you have trouble visualizing the size of an inflamed area that someone else describes as 4 cm?

One way to take the guesswork out of such situations is to have everyone use a standard chart for reference. The chart used in labor and delivery to measure cervical dilatation is ideal. Simply display the chart where it's accessible to the entire unit staff and have them refer to the chart for assessment of wound drainage or measurement of any area up to 10 cm in size.

The use of such a chart makes charting simpler and more consistent, and saves time in shift reports.

—MARY S. HALL, RN

NO OVERFLOW WOES

When a fracture pan overflows, changing the bed linens can be painful for your patient. But you can easily prevent such overflow by siphoning urine away from the fracture pan. Here's how.

Get some straight tubing, a 30-cc syringe, and a urine collector. Place one end of the tubing into the fracture pan, the other end onto the syringe's needle. Position your patient on the pan and place the urine collector at a lower level.

As the patient starts to void, pull the syringe's plunger back. This will create suction and start a flow of urine. Remove the syringe from the tubing, and quickly place the tubing into the collector.

Besides reducing your patient's discomfort, this technique will reduce your hospital's linen usage. You can also use the technique when giving perineal care.

—LINDA HOOKER, RN

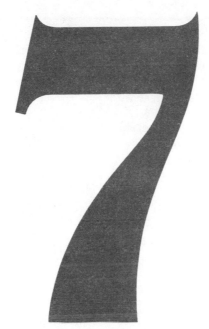

Caring for pediatric patients

EVERYBODY WINS

If you do skin tests on children, make the testing less traumatic by using this guessing game.

First, divide the child's back into sections according to the different types of allergens (weeds, trees, and so on). Next, ask both the child and his parent to guess how many allergy extract drops you'll administer in each section.

Then, as you administer the drops, count them. If someone guesses the exact number, he gets two points. If neither parent nor child guesses correctly, the player with the closest guess gets one point. The player with the highest score wins. Repeat the game for each section of the child's back, until the allergy testing is complete.

The game lets the child relax between administrations and diverts his attention from the test. The few minutes you spend explaining the game beforehand save many minutes of fighting, crying, and struggling. So, really, everyone— child, parent, and you—wins.

—BEVERLY OPITZ, RN

EASIER POSTURAL DRAINAGE

When parents have to perform daily postural drainage and percussion on a young child with cystic fibrosis, suggest they get a bean bag chair for their home.

Using this chair, they can easily place a child in several comfortable positions. As a bonus, the smaller chairs are often decorated with cartoons and bright colors, which children like.

—SHARON BEAN, LPN

BRIGHT SIGHTS

Keep a large, brightly painted wooden animal propped against the wall in each pediatric room. The puppies, frogs, bears, and other creatures delight patients. But—more important—they make an easily accessible board to place beneath a child during a code.

—KAREN PASLEY, RN

IN A SPIN

How can you encourage a child who has just had surgery or who has a respiratory disease to do his breathing exercises? Give him a simple pinwheel toy which spins as the child blows on it. It's good for him, and fun, too.

—VICKI LUTTERELL, RN, BSN

HUGGING MOMMY

Here's a way to make preoperative injections less traumatic for young children, and for you, too. Have the child sit on his mother's lap and hug her while you're giving the injection. Hugging mommy gives the child a feeling of security and keeps his muscles relaxed while you're inserting the needle. If the child begins to fight back, his mother simply hugs him tighter. This is much nicer than having strangers hold the child while he's getting his injection.

—PHYLLIS A. SMITH, RN

RACK THEM UP

Where to keep toothbrushes and toothpaste in a school building could be a problem.

A solution is to cement together 7-inch (17.5-cm) lengths of 2-inch-wide (5-cm-wide) plastic pipe, which you can get from a plumber, to make

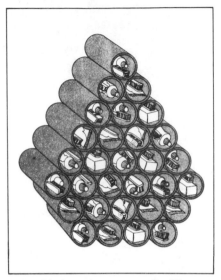

pyramid-shaped storage racks. The students can store their supplies hygienically inside a piece of pipe. Putting a rack inside each rest room, will cut down on students' traveling time.

Spray each rack with bright heat-resistant acrylic enamel paint. And increase the storage space at any time by cementing more lengths of pipe to the racks.

—CYNTHIA A. MARMEN, RN

SMALL IS BETTER

Getting toddlers to increase their fluid intake can be a real problem, as you know. One solution is to offer small amounts of fluid in a 1-ounce (30-ml) medicine cup. The cup doesn't intimidate the patient as much as a large drinking glass would, and the child will more readily sip a teaspoon or two of fluid.

By offering the cup frequently, you can substantially increase your patient's daily fluid intake. Also, since the cup is premeasured, keeping an accurate record is simple.

—URSULINE FERGUSON, RN

BIRTH-DAY MEMENTO

Here's a good-bye gift for new parents.

When the parents leave with their baby, give them a special page for their baby book. The page, made up of newspaper clippings from the day the baby was born, includes front-page headlines, food and fashion ads, and astrology and weather reports.

—MARY EGGEN, RN

PICTURE PRIDE

Give pediatric patients crayons and paper and ask them to draw self-portraits while they wait to see the doctor. When finished, they can hang their pictures on a picture board—a bulletin board on the waiting room wall.

This activity keeps young patients busy, and they're proud of their contributions to the waiting room's decor.

—TONI PILLER, RN

LET'S PRETEND

Trying to get a 2-year-old to take medicine can be a real battle. Before he has to take antibiotics or cough medicine, pretend to give some to a doll. After watching a "sick" dolly take the medicine, the child will happily take his dose.

—PATRICIA TREFETHEN, RN

CAP IT OFF

When children have a sutured laceration on the scalp with a dressing that needs to be kept clean, use a bathing cap. Choose one that's a size larger than needed, and it will keep the bandage clean and secure. The caps come in decorative colors so children can pretend they're airplane pilots with their rubberized headgear.

—ANN CUNNINGHAM, RN

KEEPSAKE COPY

As a special memento for new parents, make another copy of the baby's footprints for them. The footprint form also has space to list the baby's vital statistics—birth weight, length, time of birth, and so on. On the other side, use a rubber stamp to record visiting hours, mother's room number, and phone numbers.

Not only do parents appreciate the keepsake copy, but you're spared having to repeat the same information over and over, so it's a timesaver for you.

—MARYANN MCNAMARA, RN

CIRCUITOUS SOLUTION

Getting small children to force fluids can be a problem. Use plastic "crazy straws," which are constructed in complicated shapes. The youngsters love watching the path of the juice when they sip. They take adequate fluids and won't let the straw out of sight.

—DIANNE CHARRON, RN

MINIATURE URINAL

How many times have you used a urine collection bag on a premature male infant, only to have the bag slip off the infant's penis?

Here's a more effective urine collector: a capped syringe, with the needle and plunger removed.

After inserting the infant's penis

through the syringe's open end, place a strip of hypoallergenic tape over the closed end. Then, tape the syringe to the infant's lower abdomen or groin.

With this miniature urinal, you don't lose any of the infant's urine sample. So you get enough urine for testing, and you can measure intake and output accurately. Also, you can see the penis through the clear, plastic syringe, to check for pressure.

—NANCY J. URICH, RN, BS

SOAKING SOLUTION
When burn wounds or infected cuts on an active toddler's hand or fingers need to be soaked several times a day, how do you gain his cooperation? Try placing brightly colored, nonfloating objects or large coins on the bottom of the soaking basin. Then challenge the toddler to reach into the warm solution and bring them out. He may have trouble grasping some of the objects or he might drop them before getting them out of the solution, but this will prolong the soaking time.

When he has all the objects out, ask him to place them back on the bottom again. Although this method takes longer to achieve the desired soaking time, it keeps the toddler interested.

—ROSE ALAYNE WILKERSON, RN

"BABY-GRAMS" FOR PARENTS
If babies in the neonatal intensive care unit are brought in from rural areas, their parents have to travel long distances to visit or else make expensive phone calls.

Keep parents posted on their baby's progress by sending "baby-grams" on inexpensive postcards. On the card's message side, put the baby's footprint and a short note "from the baby."

The note can state the baby's weight and say something positive about his condition, if only to describe his curly hair or lusty cry. Parents love getting these cards and can add them to their baby books.

—NANCY HOGG, RN

SCHOOL SLEUTHS
If you're a school nurse, teach the home economics and physical education teachers how to spot shoulder and hip disproportions—locker rooms and sewing classes are ideal places to spot scoliosis.

—SHERRY FRENCH, RN

CUDDLY CAPS
Make stocking caps for the babies in an intensive care nursery. Since the babies' greatest heat loss is from their heads, the caps help keep their temperatures stable, decreasing their caloric needs. Also, the caps seem to make parents less preoccupied with the monitoring equipment, and more aware of their babies' normal aspects.

—DIAN LOOMER, RN
LINDA MacKENZIE, RN

HOW DRY I AM
Advise new mothers on how to promote umbilical cord healing, and how to treat diaper rash. Getting plenty of air to the area being treated is an important part of the healing process, and a handheld blow-dryer works perfectly. Set the dryer on "warm," and hold it 6 to 8

inches from the skin for 5 minutes four times a day. Besides helping to heal the skin, the warm air may lull the babies into a quiet state.

—BARB PRIOR, RN

QUICK-COOLING GAUZE

Here's an easy way to bring down a child's elevated temperature.

First, remove the padding inside a 4x4 gauze pad, leaving the wide-gauge gauze. Soak this gauze in lukewarm water. Then, place the wide-gauge gauze over the child's abdomen, wrists, and ankles, and rewet the gauze every few minutes.

This technique brings a child's temperature down more rapidly than sponging or using heavy rags and cloths.

—CYNTHIA SUNDMAN, RN

PERCUSSION DISCUSSION

For an effective, reusable infant chest percussion tool, tape a *plastic* medicine cup (a paper cup weakens after one or two uses) to the end of a tongue blade. Cushion the blow with a cotton ball taped to the edge of the cup.

Ordinary plastic nipples can also be used for infant chest percussion. They're safe, soft, and, with the base trimmed a bit, small enough to use on tiny and premature infants. They work especially well if you have to percuss between monitor leads on a tiny chest.

—MARY WALKER, RN

INJECTION QUESTION

Remembering to rotate injection sites can be difficult for young diabetics. Turn this problem into a game by cutting out a large, cardboard doll, and marking the injection sites on the doll's arms, legs, and abdomen. On the back of the doll, draw a chart with the various sites on the left, and the days of the week across the top. Every time a patient gives himself an injection, he checks

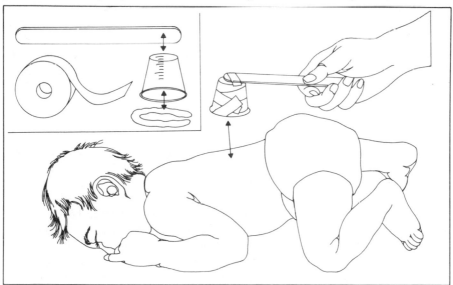

off the site under the appropriate day. And you need only check the doll to see where the next injection should be given.

—E. WEINSTOCK, RN

PUT UP A HAPPY FACE

To increase visual stimulation for infants who require restraint (such as those undergoing cleft lip repair), tape pictures of happy, smiling faces inside their cribs. Toothpaste advertisements in magazines are especially good, and the little ones seem to enjoy gazing at human faces.

—RITA A. FLEMING, RN

COLLECTING URINE SPECIMENS

Here's how to collect a 24-hour urine specimen from an infant without using a catheter.

First, cleanse the infant's perineal area and let it dry completely. Then attach a 3- or 4-inch (7.5- or 10-cm) square piece of Stomahesive to a 24-hour collection bag. Cut a center hole in the Stomahesive and contour the edges to fit the baby's perineal area.

Next, remove the backing from the Stomahesive and moisten the Stomahesive with water to attach it to the baby's perineal area. The baby's body heat helps seal the adhesive, so hold the bag in place for a few seconds. (And for better adhesion, if the baby is a boy, place his penis *and* scrotum inside the bag.) For additional security, put nonallergenic tape around the edges.

Check the bag frequently and empty it into a jar.

Or, if you don't want to use adhesive

tape on an infant, try this:

Make two small vertical slits in the Stomahesive—one on each side of the center hole—but don't remove the paper backing. Insert a piece of twill or trach tape through each slit. Then place the bag on the baby and tie it in place around his waist—just tight enough to be secure.

—BEV PETRITES, RN

STARRED CHARTS

When pediatric patients take their prescribed medications for the day, help them see stars. Stars on their medication charts, that is.

To make a chart, take a sheet of paper, print the patient's name on it, and list his prescribed medications down the left side. Then print the days of the week across the top of the page and rule in the necessary columns. When the patient takes his medications, put an adhesive-backed star in that day's space.

Giving stars as a reward really encourages patients to take their medications. And to encourage at-home compliance, give the chart to the child's parents when he leaves the hospital.

—BRIAN J. J. COLE, SN

SOCKS TO SWIM IN

To prevent children with spina bifida from scraping their feet against a swimming pool's side or bottom, put terrycloth tennis socks on the children's feet before they go into the pool. This way they can splash to their hearts' content without scraping their feet. What's more, the socks don't interfere with the pool's filtering system.

—PAT HUNTER, RN

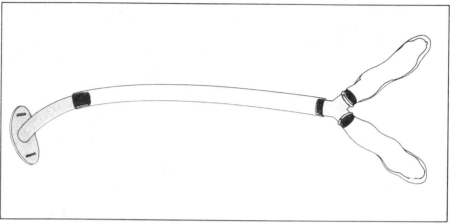

TEACHING VENTILATION

If a baby on your unit has a tracheostomy and occasionally needs artificial ventilation when he becomes apneic and stimulation won't arouse him, you'll need to teach his mother how to ventilate him at home.

To help her practice, make a model respiratory system from the following materials: two finger cots, two rubber bands, a small Y-connector, some oxygen tubing, and a trach tube. Use the Y-connector to attach the finger cots to the oxygen tubing, securing them with the rubber bands. Then, attach the trach tube to the other end of the tubing. Finally, attach an Ambu bag to the trach tube.

Now the mother can practice gauging the amount and rate of pressure needed to inflate the finger-cot "lungs." When she becomes proficient in ventilating the model, she can take the baby home.

—J. THUMAN, RN

THROW IN THE TOWEL

To get a 24-hour urine specimen from a newborn baby girl, place a rolled-up towel between the baby's knees and ankles, attaching it to her legs with 2-inch (5-cm) paper tape. When her legs are separated (as if she had a hip-spica cast), the urine bag can be taped on securely, and she can't kick it out of place. Also, the baby can easily be turned from her back to her stomach.

—JOAN M. MOORE, RN, MN

THE KIT'S A HIT

A "Mother's Sick Child Care Kit" will save you from dashing to the grocery store for clear liquids and diversional activities when your children are sick. Use a brightly colored tote bag and fill it with packages of gelatin, powdered fruit drinks, crackers, tissues, a can of soft drink, a thermometer, children's aspirin, some crayons, and a coloring book.

Give these kits as gifts (they can be modified for children of different ages) to friends and patients so they'll be prepared the next time one of their children comes down with the flu or some other common childhood illness.

—SHANNON PATTON, RN

DIAPER LIFT

Ever care for a young child who had a hernia repair and circumcision? Pressure irritates his penis and he can't wear a diaper—at least not in the regular fashion.

So to keep him dry *and* comfortable, take an 8-ounce (240-ml) paper cup and devise a penis cradle for him. After removing the cup bottom, slit the cup in four places: two slits in the front and

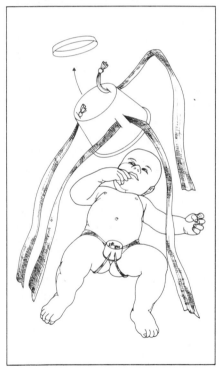

one on either side. Then cut four long gauze pieces, thread one piece through each slit, and knot the ends inside the cup so they won't pull out.

Next, put the cup over the child's penis, with the cup front facing his buttocks. After bringing the two side gauze pieces around the child's waist and the

front pieces up from under his buttocks, tie all four together at his back like a belt. Finally, put a diaper on the child *over the cup*.

By lifting the diaper up, the cup keeps pressure off the child's penis. Yet the diaper "does its duty" and helps keep the child's clothes and bed dry.

—JAMIE L. HAFER, LPN

EDIBLE ICE BAG

If you're a pediatric or public health nurse, here's a tip you can pass on to parents of small children.

Next time Junior bumps his head (or leg or arm), don't waste time finding a towel and filling a plastic bag with ice cubes. Instead, just reach for a bag of frozen vegetables from your freezer and apply it to the injured area.

Suggestion: If by chance you've grabbed Junior's favorite vegetable, promise to let it thaw and serve it to him for dinner.

—M. LORRAINE STEWART, RN

ROAD BED

How can you keep the pediatric patient on complete bed rest occupied? After the novelty of new coloring books wears off, the child longs for an action game. Some paper towels—plus imagination—make the perfect answer for a little boy who loves playing with model cars.

Laying eight to ten paper towels end to end, tape them together and draw a "road" down the middle. After cutting out the road, encourage the boy to add his own twists—e.g., passing zones, curves, and so on. The young road designer will contentedly drive his toy cars up and down pillow mountains and through blanket tunnels for hours.

—SALLY GOODHART, LPN

GET A GRIP ON IT

The barrel of a plastic syringe makes a nice hand-grasp exerciser for unresponsive children.

Remove the plunger from the syringe, cover the end of the barrel with tape, and place the barrel in the child's hand. It's narrow enough for the small hand and fingers to grasp, yet wide enough to prevent the child from clenching and embedding his fingernails into his palm. (A 3-ml syringe usually fits the grasp of children to age 2; a 10-ml syringe fits most older children.) But to avoid a contracture, remove the exerciser for 2 hours after every 2 hours of use.

—MARIAN SWIST, RN

THROAT SOAK

Children with sore throats don't always take their cough syrups and fluids as prescribed, so their recovery is prolonged.

To speed up the healing process, offer them warm gelatin desserts to drink. Although they're not a substitute for cough syrups, they help promote comfort and recovery. They coat the throat, relieve soreness, provide necessary fluids, and—best of all—they come in many popular flavors.

—CAROL WILT, RN, BSN

BABY KEEPSAKE

Many infants in a neonatal unit need to have an intravenous tube inserted into a scalp vein at one time or another. Already worried about the newborn's illness, the parents become upset about having their baby's head shaved.

To allay the parents' anxieties (especially for the first shaving), tape the infant's shaved hair to a card listing his name, age, weight, and the date.

Besides letting them know that you understand their concern, the card is a nice baby keepsake for the parents.

—NANCY HOGG, RN

HELP FOR HANDICAPPED TOTS

To help a handicapped toddler learn to walk, make a set of sturdy, economical parallel bars from wooden dowels and ordinary kitchen chairs.

At a lumber company, buy two 8-foot dowels, 1 inch in diameter. Sand and varnish the dowels and attach a piece of clothesline rope to each end with a small nail. Then place the dowels over

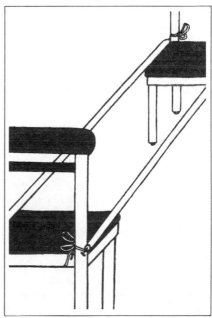

the seats of two kitchen chairs and tie the ends of the dowels to the chair backs. The height and width of the chair seats is just right for a toddler.

When the bars aren't in use, untie them and put them away.

—HELEN HOKE, RN

MEDI-MINDER

An infant with cardiac problems requiring at-home drug therapy obviously must depend on his parents to follow through.

To simplify compliance, give parents a monthly open-block calendar. In each daily block, ask them to list the infant's prescribed drugs and their administration times. After administering each dose, the parents should check off the time administered.

Be sure to advise parents to fill out only a week's worth of blocks at a time, because their doctors might add to or discontinue the regimen. Also suggest they not list doses, because these, too, could be changed. Instead, supply a small card listing the dosage for each drug, which can be kept with the drugs for handy reference.

The calendar really helps parents organize and keep track of their infant's multiple prescriptions. As a result, it's a real spur to parent compliance—and to infant good health.

—ANNE L. McKINNON, RN, BSN

BABY ALARM

When a baby goes home with a tracheostomy, his parents usually worry about how they'll know if he wakes up at night, since he can't cry. Suggest they get some tiny jingle bells—the kind tod-

dlers wear on their shoes—and string them on ribbons to tie around the baby's wrist or ankle. Double-knotting the bells ensures that they won't come off so the baby won't swallow them.

Parents report that these "alarm bracelets" help *them* sleep better at night—at least until they hear the bells jingle.

—CRAIG UHLER, RN, USN

COUNTERING *CANDIDA*

When a baby has thrush, lactose in his formula or his mother's milk can promote the growth of *Candida albicans*. To prevent such growth, advise the mother to rinse her baby's mouth with water after each feeding.

—BETH L. HAUG, RN

DISAPPEARING INK

The footprinting and fingerprinting procedure in the delivery room leaves hard-to-remove ink stains on baby and mother. But with some gauze dabbed in a bit of baby oil, cleanup is easy. Just wipe the stains with the gauze and the ink will disappear—in a jiff.

—JACKIE ANGLE, RN, BSN

PAGING IN THE E.D.

To keep a frightened child occupied while he's waiting to be examined in the emergency department (ED), give him an "activity page" and a box of crayons. On one side of the page include drawings and descriptions of objects and people he'll see in the ED. On the other side include spaces in which to write his name, his doctor's and nurse's names, and the reason he came to the ED. Also offer a connect-the-dots drawing of a child with a broken leg and crutches.

Besides giving children something to do, these activity pages introduce them to the ED in a pleasant, nonthreatening way. And parents think they're a better reward than candy.

—GINGER KROPP, LPN

STOCKED UP

When a patient arrives on the neonatal ICU, set up a medication box for him. But if medications must be started immediately—before you can stock the box, try this.

Instead of borrowing medications or waiting for the pharmacy to fill the prescription, take medications from your stock supply. Keep a card for each stock medication in the same drawer.

To keep track of which medications should be charged to which patients, place an appropriate card from the stock drawer in the patient's medication box. Then, when the pharmacy sends the patient's prescribed drugs to the unit, take the card from the patient's box and return it, with the medication, to your stock drawer.

—NANCY GANC, SN

A TRACE OF FUN

Make body tracings for young diabetics to teach them proper rotation of insulin injection sites.

Trace the child's body outline on brown wrapping paper. The two sides of the paper represent the front and back of his body. After each injection, help the child find and date the site on the paper.

Children can decorate the tracings

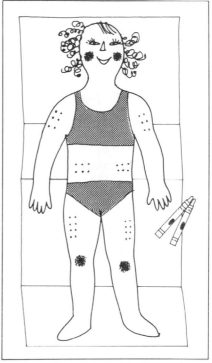

with yarn, felt-tip pens, and other supplies available on your unit. When discharged, they can take the artwork home for continued use.

—ANN EMERY, RN, BSN

UPSIDE-DOWN SHIRT

Disposable diapers with plastic covers are great time-savers in an intensive care nursery. But they can create problems, too—like chafed babies' bottoms. Exposing the affected areas to the air will speed healing, but the babies may get cold.

Solve the chafing problem, and keep the babies' temperature stable by putting long-sleeved infant shirts on the babies when you expose them to air. Their legs go through the sleeves, and their bottoms stick through the neck openings—keeping everything covered except the affected areas. Mothers like the way their babies look, too.

—SUE LEONARD, RN

NUTRITION RUMMY

To encourage children to select from the four basic food groups and avoid junk foods, use a card game to teach them sound nutrition principles.

To play the game, you need 52 playing cards, color coded according to food groups and divided as follows:

- 10 *milk-group* cards (black borders)
- 10 *cereal-group* cards (blue borders)
- 10 *fruit/vegetable-group* cards (green borders)

(Each of these groups has five cards labeled for one serving and five labeled for two servings.)

- 10 *meat-group* cards (red borders), all labeled for one serving

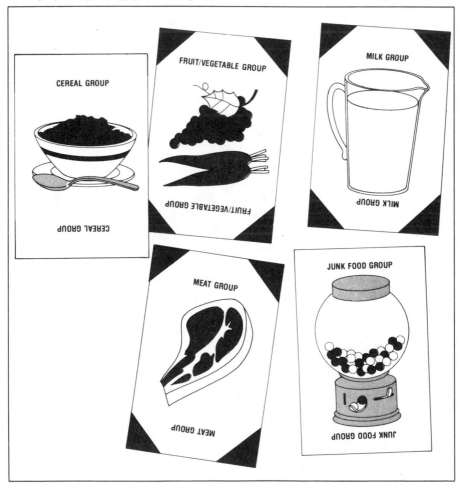

• 12 *junk-food* cards with one picture on each (e.g., popcorn, candy, cookies, gum).

To make the playing cards, cut 3x5 cards into 2¼x3½-inch (5.7x8.7-cm) pieces. Then label each card, color in its border, and paste on an appropriate magazine picture.

Before the children start the game, make sure a "Guide to Good Eating" poster from a local dairy or nutrition center is hanging close by. The poster will guide the children as they play, especially regarding the servings suggested for each food group. Once the game begins, it's played just like rummy.

Two to four players are dealt 11 cards each. The remaining cards are placed face down, except for the top card, which the dealer turns over to begin a discard pile. Each player then draws the top card from the face-down pile or the discard pile.

The player then discards one card, so he doesn't have more than 11 cards after his turn. The first player to lay down 10 or 11 cards with the correct number of servings in each food group wins the game. For example, a winning hand might have two 1-serving and one 2-serving fruit/vegetable cards, one 1-serving and one 2-serving milk cards, four 1-serving cereal cards, and two 1-serving meat cards.

To test the game's effectiveness, give the children a nutrition quiz before the game. Then see if the children answered more questions correctly *after* playing.

—NANCY MATHESON, RN

SEE AND SAW

To help children in Halo-Tibial traction watch TV or even see around the room, use a car clip-on mirror. Not only can it be swivelled in any direction but it fits perfectly on the bars of the traction.

—CHERYL IZENOUR, RN

PUPPET PAL

Getting a young patient to sit still for 20 minutes while his hand soaks in povidone-iodine (Betadine) solution can be an ordeal. So turn the treatment into a game.

Soak some 4x4 bandages in a Betadine solution, apply them to the laceration, and then slip your patient's hand into an examination glove to keep the 4x4s in place. Using a marking pencil, draw eyes, a nose, and a mouth on the glove, creating a hand puppet. After this your patient looks forward to his next treatment—and a new puppet pal.

—LYNN BROESCH, LVN

TALES OF DISTRACTION

Suturing a minor laceration or changing a dressing on a squirming child is always a challenge. Rather than use sedatives or restraints to keep him still, try to enlist the child's cooperation with story-telling and a reward.

If you rarely have a person available just to stand by and read a story, tape some children's favorites on cassettes. After you explain the procedure, the child chooses a story, and puts the proper cassette in the player. Then, instead of concentrating on his discomfort, the child becomes engrossed in the story.

When you finish the procedure, blow up a rubber glove, tie a knot at the cuff, draw a face on it with a felt-tip marker, and give the child the "balloon." This reward is simple, inexpensive, and appealing.

—CAPT. SUSAN B. SHIPLEY, RN

KEEPING SCORE

To encourage pediatric patients to take fluids after surgery, devise an attractive "scorecard."

Draw on a sheet of paper various symbols representing fluids: soda bottles, Popsicles, ice cream, Jell-O, milk,

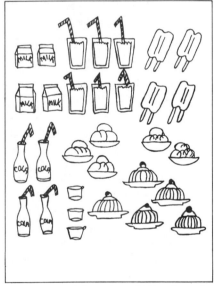

and water. After the child takes the fluid, he colors the appropriate symbol on his scorecard.

—MARTHA CLARK, RN

CAST OFFS

"When is my cast coming off?" is a question pediatric patients ask repeatedly. But since many patients have only a vague concept of time, invent a visual aid to help them count the days: calendar cards.

Number a set of cards—one card for each day the child has to wear his cast—and hang them above his bed, like a mobile. The patient can remove one card each day, and see the numbers get smaller, or can count the remaining cards to see how many days are left.

As the number of cards decreases, the number of smiles increases!

—LINDA WYSZINSKI, RN

CROSS OFF THE PILL

Don't worry about whether parents give their children's medications properly. Instead, create a visual aid for parents—a cross-off-the-pill chart. Each chart should have 10 boxes—one for each day of the antibiotic course. Inside each box, write "1, 2, 3, 4" to designate the number of pills to be taken each day. Have the patient simply cross off a number after each pill he takes. On the flip side of the chart, list general instructions for taking antibiotics.

Now, patients can hang up their charts in a prominent place, remind their parents when they need a pill, and cross off the numbers themselves.

—PHYLLIS YETKA, RN

AN EASY WEIGH

Standard baby scales are usually too small for large or handicapped young patients. Adult scales aren't much better; they're often imprecise (especially at lower weights) and are inadequate for handicapped children who can't stand on the base of the scale.

As pictured here, a "bathtub swing scale" can hang on a door frame with the clamp from a baby's jumping exerciser. Place a hanging scale (available

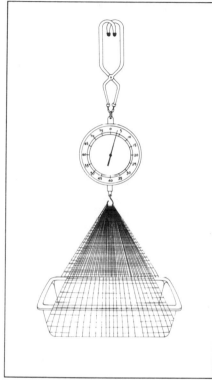

from feed stores) on the clamp, and attach a fishnet-hammock—which you can find in a boating or sporting goods store—to the bottom of the scale. Finally, place a plastic baby's bathtub in the hammock to assure smooth sailing during the weigh-in.

The scale is lighter, less expensive, and more easily dismantled and transported than the typical baby and adult scales.

—BARBARA CHEYNEY, RN, PHN

DOWN THE SPOUT

Getting bedridden patients to drink used to cause more fluid spilled than consumed, especially with tots who haven't quite mastered drinking through straws, or postop patients who aren't allowed straws. Eliminate the mess by using special drinking cups—the kind that have a snap-on lid with a spout in it. They can be found in most grocery stores or drugstores. So, if a patient can raise his head, he can drink—unassisted and unafraid of spilling.

—DIANE VOELLNER, RN, MN

REGULAR CHECKUPS

If you're a school nurse, checking expiration dates on vaccines and medications can be a tedious job. But it's a job that has to be done regularly.

To make the checking easier and less tedious, post a 3-year chart in your injection room. The chart has a space for each month say from January, 1983, to December, 1985. When a new vaccine or medication comes in, record its expiration date in the appropriate month. Since you can see at a glance what medications will be outdated the next month, reordering is easier, too.

—H. IRENE MILLER, RN

BOUNCY MOBILE

Here's a way to make a colorful, inexpensive mobile to stimulate infants and bedridden youngsters. Punch eight holes in a paper or Styrofoam dinner plate, making a circular pattern. Cut a long piece of string into four, 24-inch (61-cm) pieces, then thread each piece up through the bottom of the plate and down through the next hole.

Now you can be creative. Cut animal pictures from magazines, or make snowflakes or other shapes from colored paper, and tie your creations to the strings hanging from the plate. To suspend the mobile, just punch two more holes in the center of the plate, and thread a strong rubber band through the holes, tying it to a long string at the top. Then tape the string to the ceiling or hang it from the I.V. pole.

The rubber band makes the animals and snowflakes dance if the child pulls on the mobile, and gives the plate some bounce so it won't tear easily.

—SYLVIA SPEARR, RN

CHILDREN ONLY, PLEASE

Do you use oversized wheelchairs or large carts to transport children from the pediatrics unit to other areas of the hospital? This often adds to their fright in unfamiliar surroundings.

To make this experience as pleasant as possible, use a large red wagon that comfortably carries children up to the age of about 9. Since most children have a wagon at home, it gives them something to relate to and makes their trip a happier experience.

—BARBARA BERGER, RN
BARBARA JURGELIS, RN

FEEDING EASY

Feeding a baby with a cleft palate can be discouraging for a new mother—even when using a commercial cleft palate nipple. But if you put a small slit through the hole of a regular nipple, the baby can feed easily.

Tell the mother to place the nipple into the baby's mouth with the slit in a vertical position. Make sure the nipple's angled so the baby's tongue and existing palate can compress it.

Although the baby can't form a vacuum to suck, he'll work at the nipple and cause the slit to open and close to produce a flow of milk.

Remind the mother to hold her baby in an upright position while feeding him. He'll also need to be burped more often than babies who suck normally.

This simple "nipple-slit" allows mothers and babies to enjoy feeding time together—a real boon for both.

—NANCY FINNEGAN, RN

PADDING THE PREEMIE

Occasionally, an unswaddled, over-zealous premature infant will rub his knees, elbows, toes, and even his chin against his bed linens, causing painful abrasions. To protect these delicate areas, apply small karaya pads to his skin.

When moistened, the pads adhere, making a soothing barrier against harsh linens. And removal is easy: The pads come off in one piece without pulling the skin.

—MICHELE DAWSON, RN, BS

EXIT ENNUI

Boredom and short attention spans are problems in pediatrics.

Use a "Game Crash Cart" filled with cards, crayons, books, tracing paper, puppets and other toys liked by both boys and girls of all ages.

The gaily decorated cart creates an air of excitement and joy for bedridden patients. It's an orderly way of keeping many diversionary objects available for the children.

—JOANNE SERAPILIA, SN

SHOW AND TELL

Explaining a procedure before doing it is just as important with children as it is with adults. But, if a very young child can't understand a verbal explanation, try drawing a picture.

You needn't be a great artist—stick figures will serve the purpose very well. Show the child what will happen as you explain the procedure to him.

The picture also serves as a distraction while you're actually doing the procedure. The child can compare the real equipment with the picture you've drawn for him.

—SANDRA DEWULF, RN

MED TRAYS MADE FUN

Those plastic trays sometimes sold at fast-food restaurants can double as medicine trays for pediatric patients. They're durable, inexpensive, stackable, and have spaces for drinking cups, med icine cups, and syringes.

Best of all, the trays are brightly decorated with the fantasy, TV, and movie characters popular among children. And a familiar face (even if it *is* on a medicine tray) can do much to make a youngster more comfortable with unfamiliar hospital routines.

—DONNA MAHEDY, RN, PNP

HUNGRY HOUND

Use flash cards and a toy dog to teach nutrition basics to first, second, and third graders.

To make the cards, you'll need the following:
- a 20x54-inch (50x135-cm) cardboard sheet
- 36 magazine pictures of junk foods and foods from the four basic food groups
- glue or paste.

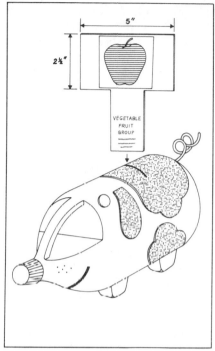

Measure and cut the cardboard into 36 5x6-inch (12.5x15-cm) pieces, then cut each piece into the shape of a "T," 5 inches (12.5 cm) wide and 6 inches (15 cm) high (see illustration). Glue a food picture on the T's horizontal bar. On the vertical bar, print the name of the food group(s) represented by the picture and the words "Healthy for You" or "Not Healthy for You."

To make the dog, you'll need these materials:
- 1 empty gallon bleach bottle with cap
- 1 empty egg carton
- black or brown pipe cleaner
- black and brown felt
- glue.

Cut four rounded egg holders out of the egg carton. Glue them to one side of the bottle to represent his feet—and to enable the bottle to stand.

Cut out three small black felt disks. Glue two of them into position as eyes; glue the third to the bottle cap for the nose.

Cut two pieces of brown felt in the shape of long, floppy ears, and glue these to the bottle sides.

Bore or punch a hole into the bottom of the bottle, and slide the pipe cleaner into the hole. Twist the pipe cleaner to make a curly tail.

Set the bottle on its feet and cut a 2⅛-inch (5.3-cm) slit into the top. You—or the children—can give the dog felt spots or decorations if you like.

To play the game, slide a T card into the dog's top so that only the food picture shows. Ask the children to name the food shown and to tell whether it's a junk food or to which food group it belongs. Pull the card out of the slot to check answers.

Children can play this game by themselves, in pairs, or as a class. But however they play it, they're sure to have fun *and* to learn about the foods they eat.

—LESLIE GRANO, RN

DISPOSAMOBILE

Use a disposable face mask to make a mobile for a crib-bound infant in an intensive care or isolation unit.

Tie a favorite rattle, small toy, or even a colorful hospital bootee to two tie strings of a face mask. Secure the other two tie strings to the cross bars of the crib.

The "mobile" is sturdy enough to last several days, but you can change the toys more often to provide new stimuli for the infant.

—KATHRYN WHEAT, RN

TINY TONGUE BLADE

You may have trouble examining the mouth of a newborn—a tongue blade, even a junior one, is too big for the tiny patient's mouth.

Use the *handle* end of a cervical scraper as a tongue blade. Because it's only half the width of a conventional blade, it ends problems with oral exams.

—GALE B. JOHNSTON, RN

EGG ROLES

Those plastic egg-shaped containers for panty hose can help your adolescent and pediatric patients beat the hospital blahs. For example, have the older children make small toys for the younger ones. They can put a wooden spool or similar object inside a container, glue the halves together, and decorate them with decals. Or, adolescents can create attractive cradle mobiles by punching holes at both ends of a decorated egg, then stringing several together.

To add a seasonal touch to hospital trays, let patients transform the containers into candy-filled Easter eggs or bunnies, Thanksgiving turkeys, or Christmas Santas or elves. And, of course, with a little imagination, patients can make festive Christmas-tree ornaments from the containers.

You'll find that choosing new roles for these egg containers is fun for both the adolescents who hatch the projects and the youngsters who receive the results.

—MILDRED A. FELIZ, RN

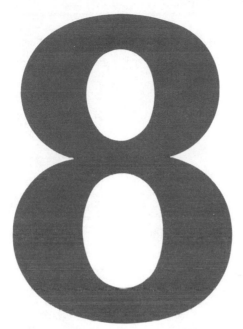

Personal appearance

POLISH PLUS

Do you find that polish alone just can't cover those black scuff marks on your nursing shoes? Try spraying the marks first with a prewash laundry spray and rubbing them with a damp cloth. Then polish as usual. They'll be clean and professional looking once again.

—Pam Hietbrink, RN

SKIRTING THE PROBLEM

One side effect of cortisone therapy is frequent up-and-down weight changes. So a patient can spend a lot of time and money buying comfortable clothes for each weight change.

To keep a female patient stylish yet solvent, get her to try wraparound skirts. They're easy to adjust and can be found on ready-to-wear racks and in pattern books. Also, depending on the style and material, a wraparound skirt is suitable for nearly any occasion.

—Karin Conway, RN

POCKET PROTECTOR

To keep pencils from smudging your uniform pockets, cover each pencil point with a rubber tip from a Vacutainer needle. The tips protect the pencil points and keep your pockets clean.

—Norka Vélez Ramos, RN

CLOSE SHAVE

If you need to shave a patient but don't have any commercial shaving cream, you *could* use plain soap and water. Often, though, this irritates the patient's skin. Instead, try this inexpensive, readily available substitute. Mix about a tablespoon of water-soluble lubricant with an equal amount of body lotion. This combination softens the beard, moisturizes the skin, and prevents irritation.

—SANDRA MEYER, RN

TEAR REPAIR

If you get a tear in your white stockings at work and can't change to a new pair, try taping them.

Just cut two pieces of white non-allergenic tape the same size. Slide one piece adhesive-side-up under the tear, then align the tear edges and affix the tape. Affix the second piece over the tear, matching edges with the first tape.

The tape keeps the hole from getting bigger and running, and it blends well with your stockings.

—SANDRA L. TURNER, RN, MEd

FIRM BACKING

Did you ever lose a name pin because it fell off your uniform unnoticed?

To prevent this, rummage through your jewelry box for the back of an earring for pierced ears. Then put your pin on as usual, but before clasping it, slide the earring back onto the pin shaft. If the clasp opens, the earring back will keep the name pin firmly attached to your uniform.

—KATHLEEN WILLIAMS, RN, CCRN

A TIP WITH TEETH IN IT

Want to add some freshness to your denture-wearing patient's smile? Just add mouthwash to the water in his dentures' storage container. Patients like the fresh taste, and if you use an antiseptic mouthwash, you can help reduce some of the bacteria.

A word of caution, though: Don't use a mouthwash that might stain the dentures.

—AUDREY STEVENSON, RN

SCUFF STUFF

When your white shoes get deep scuffs or scratches, coat the marks with white typewriter correction fluid. The fluid will fill in the scuff, permanently hiding and sealing it. And it's waterproof and durable besides.

—PAMELA R. NUMBERS, LPN

MORE SUPPORT

If your support hose aren't being very supportive, try this.

After slipping your feet and ankles into the stockings, lie down and raise your legs to at least a 45° angle. Stay in this position for a minute or two, then pull the hosiery on the rest of the way. You'll be amazed at how much more supportive your hose can be.

—SHIRLEY A. McGUIRE, RN

ON-THE-SPOT SOLUTION

Do you get ball-point pen ink spots on your uniforms? Here's a way to remove them. Wet the stained area, then pour a small amount of 70% isopropyl rubbing alcohol on the ink spots. Give the material a quick rub, and the spots will disappear.

—LUCY DALICANDRO, RN

SOFT AND CLEAN

For a quick, easy way to bathe a patient with dry skin, roll up one 6-foot-long (180-cm) towel (cut from a bolt of terry cloth—it's less expensive that way), one regular towel, and two washcloths. Wet the towels and cloths in warm water mixed with 2 ounces (60 ml) of a lanolin-based soap, then put them into a plastic garbage bag to keep them warm until you're ready to use them.

Place the large towel over the patient's body and massage gently. Use the smaller towel for back care, one washcloth for face care, and the other for perineal care.

The bath is warm and relaxing. It will help patients feel—and look—better. And because no rinsing or drying is needed, you won't irritate the patient's sensitive skin.

—DIANE LEHMKUHL, RN

COLOR THAT COLLAR

Anyone who's had to wear a cervical collar knows it's disheartening enough without having to cope with a soiled or itchy stockinette cover.

Use smooth types of knee socks in cheerful colors to coordinate the collar with the patient's clothes. After cutting off the toe and pulling the sock on over the collar (with the heel inside, next to the patient's neck), put small pins on the front, or have the patient wear scarves that also match the clothes.

Being smoother, the sock prevents irritating rashes and, most important, is a big boost to morale.

—CHLOE STEWART, LVN

PORTABLE BEAUTY PARLOR

If you've ever wanted to wash a bedridden patient's hair but couldn't find the plastic tray used for hairwashing, here's a slick substitute. And the materials to make it are always close at hand.

Open a bath blanket to its full length and roll it into a log. Fold the rolled-up blanket into a U-shape and place it inside a large plastic bag (such as those used for contaminated waste). Put the bottom of the "U" at the bottom of the bag.

Then put the bag at the head of the bed, with its open end hanging over the edge. The bag thus becomes a three-sided basin. Put a bucket on the floor

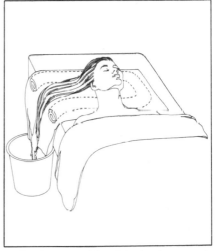

under the open side of the basin to catch the water as it drains out.

Now position the patient with his head in the basin and his neck over the rolled blanket, and scrub away. The patient will enjoy the relaxing shampoo, and you'll love the job's ease. Best of all—the bed will stay dry.

—JANICE PETERSEN, RN

MIX AND MATCH

After laundering several white pantsuit uniforms together, you may have difficulty matching the tops and bottoms correctly. Sew a small clump of colored

113

thread inside the collar and waistband, using a different color for each uniform. Then, after washing and drying, simply match the colored threads.

—ELLEN L. BADGER, RN

CLING NO MORE

Do your noncling slips persist in clinging and creeping despite your using antistatic additives in your wash? Here's a simple solution. When applying hand lotion, just wipe the excess lotion on your hose. No more will slip and skirt cling to your knees.

—BEVERLY GAULT, RN

HAIR CARE

Here's a tip for a patient with very oily hair who can't have it shampooed. Sprinkle powder through his hair. Then push the teeth of a comb through an open 4x4 and comb the patient's hair. The powder absorbs much of the excess oil, and the 4x4 collects the powder. The patient's scalp will smell cleaner. And the best part is it costs much less than dry shampoo.

—TARA HUMMEL, RN

STAIN STOPPER

Does your hospital use I.V. solutions that come in plastic bags? If so, save the small blue rubber stoppers that you remove before attaching I.V. tubing to the bags. You can use the stoppers to cap your pen and pencil points so your uniform pockets don't get stained.

—SHEILA LANGILLE, RN

REMOVES HAIR TANGLES

If you have difficulty combing tangles from patients' hair, try this: Rub the tangled strand of hair with an alcohol-saturated cotton ball, then comb. The tangles are gone and the alcohol evaporates quickly.

—IRENE EVANS, RN

POCKETS MAKE PERFECT

If your white pantsuit uniforms have no pockets in the pants, you can sew a pocket on them from any available white material. These pockets take the pressure off regular blouse pockets, which always seem to become overloaded. They also provide an excellent place to carry a notebook, tissues, scissors, keys, and whatnot. What's more, your blouse covers the pocket, so you don't have to worry about imperfections.

—RUTH THESING, RN

SPOTLESS SHOES

You know those black spots that even soap and water won't erase from your work shoes—spots that still show through the white polish? Here's a way of handling them.

Next time you clean your shoes, remove the spots first with nail-polish remover. It really works, and you'll almost believe you have new shoes.

—SUSAN KETCHAM, RN

ERADICATING LOSSES

School pins and nameplates occasionally come undone and drop off unnoticed. As a safety precaution, use a small cube of rubber, cut from an eraser.

Push the spike of your pin through the cloth of your uniform, and then slide the eraser cube onto the spike before clasping. Then, if the clasp comes undone, the cube prevents the spike from slipping through the cloth. When the cube becomes too loose, simply cut a replacement.

—VIRGINIA DAVIS, RN

HAVE A HEART

If you use telemetry to monitor cardiac patients, you know that finding a comfortable way for them to wear their transmitters can be a problem. Solve it by having heart-shaped pockets sewn on the center of the patients' gowns. The transmitters fit neatly in the pockets. An added advantage is that when cardiac patients go to other departments, such as X-ray, they can be readily identified.

—DIANE BROWN, RN

SPOT CHECK

Here's another way to get rid of those seemingly indelible ink spots that adorn your uniform pockets—the products of uncapped pen points. Just saturate the spot with hairspray, then wash your uniform with your usual detergent. The result is a truly "spotless" uniform.

—CHERYL DIORIO, LPN

ENEMA SHAMPOO

Shampooing orthopedic patients can be a challenge—especially the patients in continual traction who can't be taken to a sink. Use an "enema shampoo."

Here's how it works. Gather the following supplies: bed liners, bath towels, newspapers, a large plastic bag, a trash can or large basin, shampoo, two enema bags, and an I.V. pole. Put the head of the bed in the flat position, padding it with plenty of bed liners and towels. Spread a few newspapers on the floor and place the trash can or basin on the papers. Then cut a hole in the large plastic bag so you can slip it over the patient's head and around his neck to keep him dry. Fill the enema bags with warm water and hang them on the I.V. pole at the head of the bed.

Now have the patient hang his head over the edge of the bed and over the trash can or basin. Next, slowly release warm water from one of the enema bags over the patient's head and apply shampoo. After working it into a lather, rinse with the second enema bag. You can reuse the enema bags with as many patients as you need to, so waste can be kept to a minimum.

This procedure takes a little practice, but the patients will feel 100% better.

—SUE LOVE, RN

STAIN 'N' SCUFF PASTE

To remove ball-point pen ink from your uniforms, wet the stained area and rub in some toothpaste. Rinse, then wash your uniform as usual.

—HELEN BOSCH, RN

A HELP FOR HANDS

Giving skin and nail care to elderly patients who have contractured hands can be painful for them. Soaking hands in Vaseline first helps remove dead skin and clean under the nails with less discomfort to the patient.

Put a rubber examining glove on your own hand and coat it with Vaseline. Then pull the glove off, turning it inside out, and put it on the patient's hand. Do the same for the patient's other hand. After an hour or so, remove the gloves, wipe the patient's skin clean, and give him nail care. The softening effect of the Vaseline is a help to the patients—and to you.

—RUTH GIBSON, RN

HOW TO BEAT ACHING FEET

Do you dread having to break in a new pair of work shoes because they pinch your toes? Stuff damp washcloths in the toe of each shoe and leave them in overnight. The next day the pinch will be gone.

—PATRICIA KLEVE, LPN

WHITE AGAIN

Rust stains ruining your whites? Squeeze some lemon juice on the stains, sprinkle a generous amount of salt over the juice, and place the uniform in the sun until it's dry. Then wash as usual and—voilá!—your whites are white once again.

—ETTA M. ROSENTHAL, RN, BS, PHN

SAND DOWN TO SOFTEN UP

To soften your patient's rough heels, elbows, and knees, sand these areas lightly with *very fine* sandpaper. Then apply a liberal amount of baby oil and rub it in well. Almost instantly, even the driest, roughest skin will become soft and smooth again.

—ZOE MARGOLIS, RN, BSN

A FITTING IDEA

For a comfortable fit, don't give an obese patient *one* hospital gown—give him *two*. You'll have to do some "tailoring" first, though.

Here's how. Place the two unfolded gowns back to back and tie the neck

tapes of one gown to those of the other. Now you'll have one gown with spaghetti shoulder straps and a roomy neckline.

Put the gown over the patient's head and position one gown in front of the patient and one in the back. Then tie the lower tapes at waist level for a belted effect.

You can turn the sleeves inside out and pin them to the gown's inside, if you wish. But even if you don't, you'll probably be surprised at the gown's good—almost Grecian—look.

—ANGELA TEGARDER, LPN

SHOES LIKE NEW

Toothpaste will clean your white shoes. Just rub a dab over the scuff marks with a moist tissue or rag. Then polish with a dry tissue, and your shoes will look good as new.

—KATHY ANDERSON, RN

LOTIONED LEGS

Before putting on support hose, apply a generous amount of body or hand lotion to both your legs. And if you want to slow down absorption by the skin, mix a little glycerin with the lotion.

Either way, you'll be surprised at how much longer your hose stay up—and how comfortable they are.

—HILDA SWANSON, RN

SKIN CARE TIPS

Before shaving a male patient's beard, apply Dermassage to the stubble and leave it on for 5 minutes. This softens the beard and allows for an easy and painless shave.

—ROSE A. BRILEY, LPN

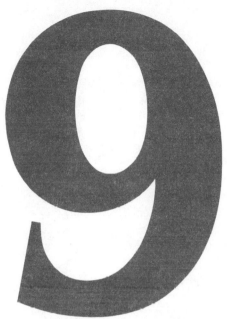

Potpourri: A medley of suggestions

TAPE REMOVER

Use a little bit of alcohol to remove adhesive tape from a patient's skin. Saturate a cotton ball with the alcohol and rub it gently over the tape and skin until the tape loosens. Then continue moving the cotton between the tape and skin until all of the tape lifts off.

—BETTY KAPANAK, RN

CHRISTMAS TREATS

Even patients on liquid diets won't have to pass up Christmas cookies—if they're made of gelatin, that is. Here's how to make them.

Combine four envelopes of unflavored gelatin with three 3-ounce (84-gram) packages of cherry- or lime-flavored gelatin. Add 4 cups (960 ml) of boiling water and stir until the gelatin

is dissolved. Pour the mixture into a 13x9-inch (32.5x22.5-cm) cookie sheet and chill until firm. Then cut out shapes with Christmas cookie cutters.

The "cookies" will help patients keep to their diets *and* enjoy some Christmas treats.

—EILEEN LAUDERMILCH, LPN

COLOR IT LARGE

To help a visually handicapped diabetic patient dip a reagent strip into his urine sample to test for sugar and acetone, make a large chart, using color swatches from a local paint store. After carefully matching each color on the bottle's chart, glue large swatches on an 8x10-inch (20x25-cm) poster board. Under each swatch, print in big letters what test result the color indicates.

117

With the color chart, the patient can perform every step in his urine test, *and* see the results.

— MARY TREVOR, RN, BSN
JERI PAYNE, NA

HANG FIRE

Hang a red envelope marked "FIRE" on each nursing unit's bulletin board. Inside the envelope put 3x5 index cards, each listing one job that should be done during a fire or fire drill (for example, "shut all doors" or "report to central dispatch"). During drills, have each staff member take one card (or more, if you're short-staffed) for her assignment.

This system reduces the "who-does-what" confusion during fire drills.

— BONNIE SHUMAKER, RN

PORTABLE STUDY AID

If you can't find the time for the study and review you need for college courses or a new job, try this method. Instead of hitting the books, hit a button—the button on a battery-operated, pocket-size tape recorder.

When you find a book or magazine article that pertains to your schoolwork or job, record its important points. Also tape the main ideas from your class notes—the notes from a one-semester course take only 3 hours to record. And if you attend a lecture that's especially interesting or helpful, the speaker's words are forever engraved on your pocket recorder.

Then, while driving to and from school and work, doing housework, or even just relaxing—you can study. And this extra time with the "books" makes you more confident on the job and more prepared for class.

— SUSAN T. ROSEN, BSN, CCRN

INSTRUMENTAL INSTRUCTION

If some employees aren't familiar with all the commonly used medical instruments, start an *Instrument of the Month* game.

First, staple a plastic instrument-holder to a manila folder. On the folder, write the name of the instrument and its pronunciation, what it's used for, and how to identify variations of the instrument. Place samples of the various instruments in the pockets of the instrument-holder. Then post the entire display on a bulletin board in the nurses' lounge.

After presenting information about hemostats, scissors, and retractors, you may notice a change for the better in the staff's handling of the instruments.

— ELLEN L. BADGER, RN

QUICK, COMFY COVER-UP

If a female patient on chemotherapy can't or won't wear a wig, she might consider this head cover-up instead.

Fold or cut a cotton scarf or piece of material into a triangle large enough to fit comfortably around the patient's head. Then, from a wig, cut a strip of hair (with its attached lining) about 1 inch (2.5 cm) wide and 4 to 6 inches (10 to 15 cm) long. (Suggestion: Cut the strip from the back of the wig; any mending here will be less noticeable.)

Center and sew the strip to the inside of the triangle's longest edge, allowing the hair to protrude like bangs. On each end of the same edge, attach a strip of Velcro tape, one inside and the other outside. When fastened together, these strips will hold the cover-up securely in place.

This cover-up will flatter the patient's face and give an illusion of hair without the bulk of a regular wig. It's great for keeping her head warm at night and handy to have around when unexpected company drops in.

—MICHELLE GRIFFIN, RN

PILLOW PRACTICE

A special pillow "abdomen" helps students practice advancing Penrose drains and removing sutures. If these procedures are included in your state's nurse practice act, you might want to try this idea, too.

To make an abdomen, cover a pillow-sized foam-rubber square with about 36 inches (90 cm) of heavy, skin-colored, synthetic suede material.

When sewing the seam, leave a 2- to 3-inch (5- to 7.5-cm) gap along one side. This allows you to replace the Penrose drain periodically.

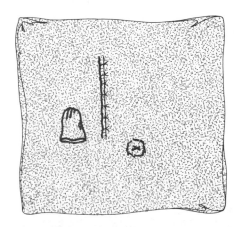

On one face of the pillow, to the left side, make a small slit through which the Penrose drain will protrude, to mimic a drain protruding from a patient's incision. To the right of this (or anywhere you wish), make a long slit— or "surgical incision"—and sew it together with silk sutures. And for atmosphere, add a belly button.

As students advance the Penrose drain through the small slit, the foam inside the abdomen offers a slight resistance, simulating actual drain advancement. Practicing this procedure and having the chance to repeatedly remove sutures helps give the students the confidence they need when they do the real thing.

—KAY SEGUNDO, RN

PADDED PULL SHEET

When you're making the bed of a bed ridden patient who needs a disposable underpad, prepare his bed as you normally would—with one exception. Instead of placing the pad on top of the pull sheet directly under the patient, sandwich it between the pull-sheet layers.

This technique will mean fewer soiled bottom sheets, thereby saving you time and cutting your hospital's linen consumption. It'll also add to your patient's comfort, because paper from the pad won't cling to his skin.

—JANET MARKEY, RN

POSTPARTUM PADS

If your postpartum patient is nursing her baby, she may appreciate this tip.

Instead of commercial bra pads, try using beltless mini sanitary pads. Simply cut a mini pad in half, peel the backing off both halves, and affix one half to each side of the bra.

The mini pad halves are highly absorbent and have a stay-dry lining that helps prevent irritated nipples and leaking. Besides, they're much cheaper—less than half the cost of most commercial bra pads.

—SUSAN LEA, RN

DOUBLE BED

If you're caring for a severely obese patient who's just too wide to turn in any hospital bed, ask the maintenance department to attach two beds and put an outer side rail on each, creating an extra-wide bed. Then, place a foam rubber "egg-crate" mattress on top of each regular mattress. To make the bed, use two regular-sized bottom sheets, and one regular-sized top sheet. Making the bed takes a few extra minutes, but the patient can turn himself quite easily.

—PAULA REES, RN

NO-FRICTION FRACTURE PAN

Before giving a fracture pan to a patient, apply some body lotion to the pan rim. The lotion will decrease the friction—and the pain—of using the pan.

—DEBORAH WOOD, RN
HELEN KELSEY, RN

GROUP THERAPY

Are you so busy that you're usually only able to give brief *individual* preoperative instructions to your patients? Supplement these individual conferences with a group session.

On the evening before their surgery, invite patients to the lounge and ask them to bring their pillows and spirometers. After discussing basic preoperative events, have the patients practice coughing and deep breathing. Also demonstrate the proper use of spirometers and how to splint incisions with pillows.

Besides ensuring that patients know what to expect the next day, the group sessions also give them the chance to share their feelings about surgery and to encourage each other.

—DONNA AVALLONE, RN

SEE HOW THEY GROW

To teach staff members the importance of infection-control practices, have them conduct a clinical experiment: making their own cultures to see how quickly bacteria grow.

First, get four agar plates. Then have the staff take cultures from their hands, the bottom of their shoes, a bedside stand, and a patient's overbed table—especially one who places used tissues on the table rather than discarding them.

After taking the cultures and labeling the plates, take them to the laboratory to be incubated for 48 hours.

Later, share the report from the laboratory. The results will show the nursing staff the importance of maintaining cleanliness.

—CHERRY A. KARL, RN, BSN

A REMOVING EXPERIENCE

Here's an easy way to remove splinters embedded under fingernails and toenails. Instead of giving your patient an anesthetic (which is often as painful as the removal itself) and cutting through the nail, file the nail's *surface* with an emery board until the nail's paper thin. Then make a small cut into the nail with an iris scissors or scalpel. The splinter will be exposed and can easily be removed with forceps.

—SUSAN B. SHIPLEY, RN, MSN

MIXES THAT MATCH

If your patient needs a dietary supplement, remember that instant breakfast mixes can substitute for drug-company supplements.

When prepared with whole milk, the mixes have nearly the same nutritional components as the supplements.

Besides, mixes are readily available in grocery stores, and even when you include the milk, they cost about half what the supplements cost. (For more protein, you can add an egg to the mix.)

Caution: Before switching from a supplement to a mix, check the labels on both to make sure the nutritional components are similar. If not, keep looking until you find a suitable match.

—DEBORAH-ANN S. COLEMAN, RN

A CLASS TIP

If you're demonstrating hemodynamic monitoring for an inservice class and want to produce some realistic wave-form patterns, try this. Just as you'd insert an inside-the-needle catheter into a vein, insert the tip of a Swan-Ganz catheter into the rubber port of a 250-ml or 100-ml bag of 5% dextrose in water. Use a large-bore needle to introduce the catheter through the rubber port.

When the catheter's in place, remove the needle, and you'll have a tight seal. Now squeeze the bag, and you'll create realistic wave-form patterns—even, with practice, dicrotic notches.

—SIGNE PRUTSMAN, RN

PUT IT ON TAPE

When your patient has an arteriovenous shunt, his cannula clamps should be easily accessible, especially in an emergency. To make sure they are, wrap a stretchy roller bandage around the patient's shunt, as usual. Then fold two

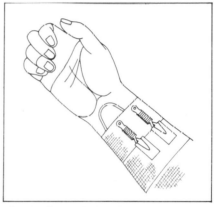

pieces of paper tape over the edge of a bandage row. Place the clamps on the paper tape.

Now you can reach for the clamps in a hurry, and they won't get stuck in the bandage's gauze fibers.

—SUE DROGOS, RN

LONG-LASTING LABEL

Do you spend a lot of time replacing the paper inserts in patients' ID bands? When the bands get wet, the information on the inserts smears.

Instead, use a labeler that punches letters on plastic strips to mark patients' names. Then slip the label (without peeling off the backing strip) into the ID band.

Although preparing these plastic strips takes a few extra minutes, the strips last much longer than the paper inserts—and that saves time and money in the long run.

—SISTER JOSEPH ANTHONY, RN

RUBBER-BAND AID

Athletic patients don't always heed warnings about resting their sprained ligaments to give them time to heal. So use a teaching aid to help them understand why proper healing takes time.

A half-inch (1.3-cm) rubber band with a small cut in the edge represents a sprained ligament in the ankle. When you stretch the rubber band, it tears even more—just as a ligament will tear if over-stretched by moving the foot.

This demonstration shows your patient how his ligament will have trouble healing unless he retires from the sporting world—for just a few days.

—ROBERT W. WOODCOCK, RN

A BRIGHT IDEA

If you're repeatedly going home from work with the narcotics cabinet keys still in your pocket, try this.

Attach the keys to one end of a long, brightly colored thick string or rope. Make a loop on the other end to slip over your head.

If the string's long enough, the keys will reach comfortably into your pocket. If it's bright enough, you'll be reminded not to take the keys home with you.

—PATRICIA DUBOVEC, RN

SHAKE-'N'-CALL

If your intensive care unit doesn't have call bells, use this way for a tracheot-omy patient to call you when he needs assistance. Place pennies or paper clips in a small, plastic, urine-specimen container. Then cap the filled container and tape it to one side rail of the patient's bed.

When the patient wants you, he just shakes his container.

—ELIZABETH MCINTYRE, BSN

REDUCING PHONE CALLS—AND ANXIETY—ABOUT HEART PATIENTS

Family visits should have a calming influence on seriously ill patients, but in many cases they have the opposite effect. One obvious reason: an anxious family transmits its anxiety to the patient.

Ask doctors what they want the families of their patients to know. Then relay that information to the family on their next visit. Or, adopt the same routine, except phone each family every morning, telling them how the patient spent the night and what the doctor had to say.

—CATHERINE BADEN, RN, BS

CHIME FOR THE NURSE

If you care for a patient who can't summon help, either by voice or call button, attach a wind chime to the I.V. standard built into the ceiling and fasten a long piece of twill tape to the chime clapper. The chime can also be attached to a regular I.V. pole. Then fasten the other end of the tape to the patient's ear with a rubber band. Thus, when the patient wants to call the nurse, he simply moves his head and the chimes ring.

The sound of the chimes is much

more pleasant than banging on the side rails or clicking the teeth or other methods that patients in similar situations usually use. Both nurses and patients appreciate it.

—MAE PAULFREY, RN, MN

WORD PLAY

To help keep up with developments in nursing, play a word game.

Every day a different person from each shift writes a new or unusual nursing-related word on the assignment sheet, and the rest of the nurses try to find out what it means.

Looking up the word takes time, but it's fun, everyone participates, and you're more likely to remember the word's meaning because you're actively searching out the word.

—BETTY HORVATH, RN

STOOL COLLECTION

To obtain stool specimens for guaiac tests from patients with bathroom privileges, give them filter paper instead of toilet paper and a stool cup to hold the paper when used. Most patients find this an easier and less offensive method of collecting stool.

—LILLIAN PLODQUIST, LPN

PICK A JOB, ANY JOB

Thanks to a "job jar," those repetitive, tedious—but necessary—tasks needed to keep the unit running smoothly can get done promptly.

Type task descriptions on separate slips of paper, fold the slips, and place them into the jar. Each nurse picks a slip from the jar, completes the designated task, and tacks the slip on the bulletin board. One nurse removes the slips from the bulletin board and recycles them as often as necessary.

Besides allowing nurses to share the load, the job jar adds an element of surprise to the unit: You never know which job you'll pick next.

—JONI L. ULMAN, RN

TODAY IS...

Here's one way to help patients with reality orientation.

Using large letters, tack the following information on the bulletin board in the general sitting area: today's weather and date (month, day, year), the facility name and city location, and the next major holiday.

Each day a patient can also announce the information over the intercom, which helps orient patients who can't read.

—MARY ZOCCHI, RN, MS

OPENING DOORS DEFTLY

Have you ever realized that opening a refrigerator door can be a problem for some patients? For instance, a patient with a fractured vertebra can't open his refrigerator door because the pulling effort causes spinal pain. To help him, suggest he use a smooth, wooden mixing paddle. Tell him to insert the edge of the paddle very gently, near the door handle, between the rubber and the refrigerator. This releases the suction, and the door will open easily.

Or try this for a patient who has rheumatoid arthritis in both hands and can't grasp the handle to open the refrigerator door. Loop an 18-inch (45-cm) piece of rope around the refrigerator handle and tie the ends together. The patient

can slip the rope over his arm to pull
the door open.

—LOUISE WIEDMER, RN, MS

BELTLESS IS BETTER

Sanitary belts with metal or plastic
hooks can cause undue pressure and
irritation to female paraplegics. Since
these patients lack sensation, they may
be unaware that an ulcerated area is
forming, especially in the sacral or coc-
cygeal areas.

So instead, use tampons or feminine
napkins with an adhesive strip that at-
taches to the undergarment.

—LOIS PINNOW, RN

NO NIGHTTIME NUISANCE

If you work nights, try this when you
make rounds. Shine the flashlight on
your white uniform. The reflected light
casts a soft glow over your patient, en-
abling you to check him without waking
him.

—P. SEIBEL, RN

SUGGESTIONS, PLEASE

Keep a suggestion box on each unit in
which nurses can deposit suggestions
for improvements in patient care. Each
week, the head nurse can review the
suggestions. Then she can list each suggestion on a flow sheet posted on the
employee bulletin board, along with a
follow-up plan of action. This provides
feedback to the nurse who made the
suggestion, so she'll know that her suggestion has actually been considered.

Not only does the system help provide better patient care, but it also helps
build good employee relations.

—LINDA KAY, RN

SHOW TIME

To familiarize new staff nurses with the
unit, give hands-on demonstrations of
various procedures with used (but clean)
equipment—Swan-Ganz catheters, fen-
estrated trach tubes, endotracheal tubes,
and so on. These show-and-tell sessions
are a welcome addition to lectures and
printed material, and they make orientation easier for the new staff and for
you.

—PAMELA STUCHLAK, RN

FLOWER HOLDER

Many times visitors arrive with cut gar-
den flowers to brighten a patient's room,
but no vases are available. Here's how
to make a substitute vase.

Take two paper cups (wax-coated or
Styrofoam), place them with mouths
together, and fasten with a strip of 1-
inch (2.5-cm) adhesive tape. Cut a hole
in one end large enough to accommodate the flower stems. Fill the vase with
water to just below the taped area. Then
add the flowers.

These vases are not only sturdy, but
also can be made in seconds from supplies kept on the floor.

—MARILEE E. HARRISON, RN

RINGS ON THEIR FINGERS

Want to know a simple trick for getting
a ring off a swollen finger? Use a few
feet of string or silk suture. Slip one
end under the ring. Beginning next to
the distal edge of the ring, wind the
other end of the string toward the fin-
gertip. The windings should be close
together to prevent the swollen tissue
from bulging through. With the coils
of string tightly in place, take the short

end of the string on the proximal side of the ring and pull it toward the tip of the finger. This pulls the ring off over the unwinding coil.

—EVANGELINE GOODWAY, RN

FOR PLASTERED ITCHES

Sticking things down into the cast to scratch itchy spots bunches up the padding and makes uncomfortable lumps. So place a hand vibrator on the cast over the itchy spot. It relieves the itching without disturbing the padding.

—DONNA HAWKINS, RN

WRISTWATCH IN ISOLATION

When working with isolation patients, do you miss being able to use your watch? Try slipping it into a plastic sandwich bag before entering the patient's room. That way you can see it, but it won't become contaminated.

—IRENE EVANS, RN

PAJAMA GAME

An irrational patient will sometimes risk traumatic injury by pulling on an indwelling urinary catheter.

Discourage this by putting a pajama bottom on the patient and running the tubing down the inside of the pajama leg. Usually, this is so successful that conventional restraints aren't necessary.

—E. REXINE STOTT, RN

ENEMA AID

The weakened rectal muscles of elderly patients often make it difficult for them to maintain a retention enema for even a short time.

To help solve this problem, administer the enema slowly. Then, roll a small towel tightly until it's about 1½ inches (3.8 cm) in diameter. Place this between the patient's buttocks against the rectum immediately after the enema is given. Have him lie on his back with the bed flat; then, the pressure of the roll will help him retain the enema.

—LOUISE WIEDMER, RN, MS

THAT OLD SMOOTHIE

You've probably heard about using a satin pillowcase to save your hairdo, but here's another idea for that old smoothie, satin.

For arthritic patients, just turning over in bed at night can be a real problem. Suggest that a satin drawsheet be made for their beds.

First, buy enough satin for the width of the bed. Then sew a strip of terrycloth or a bath towel on two ends to tuck under the mattress. Being a coarser texture, the terrycloth keeps the satin from slipping.

—ROBERTA STEELE, RN

KEEPING POSTERED

Here's a riddle: *What teaches all day, brightens a wall, and costs practically nothing?* The answer: a colorful, free brochure or poster.

Use bulletin boards to teach both patients and staff. Whenever you find an offer for a free brochure or poster in a nursing journal or family magazine, order it immediately. The materials are usually colorful, informative, and up to date. As new materials arrive, change the displays. Ordering only takes a few minutes, but the benefits last much, much longer.

—CHRISTINA M. ADDISON, RN

125

EH? SPEAK UP!

Nurses in extended care facilities frequently have problems communicating effectively with hard-of-hearing geriatric patients.

To avoid shouting yourself hoarse, place a stethoscope into the ears of the patient and talk into the bell or diaphragm. A quick wipe of the ear pieces with an alcohol sponge and the stethoscope is ready for the next patient.

—ALTA R. MILLER, RN

CAST CARE

Here's a way to help a patient protect the bottom of the foot of his leg cast from becoming broken, scraped, or dirty: Place a piece of used carpet or a carpet square over the bottom of the cast. Slash or cut out a "V-shape" at the back so the carpet fits around the heel when you bring it up toward the ankle. Hold the carpet in place with a large sock or slipper sock. Extending the carpet out beyond the toes a little will also provide some protection against bumped or stubbed toes—a welcome protection, since the toes tend to become somewhat extra sensitive to jostling.

—JUDY HUTCHINS, RN

CONTROLLED RELAXATION

The controlled-relaxation techniques for labor and delivery taught in prepared childbirth classes can be used prenatally and postpartum, too. For example, women who have difficulty falling asleep during late pregnancy may find that controlled relaxation helps induce sleep in a short time.

Also, nursing mothers who are tense or nervous at feeding times may find that controlled relaxation works just as well as a glass of wine or beer.

—MURIEL A. ZRANING, RN

TICK PICK

To remove a tick from a patient's skin, cover the tick with petroleum jelly. After a few minutes, the tick will suffocate and you can remove it painlessly with forceps.

—LINDA DELUCA, RN, BSN

JUST WHISTLE

A whistle can help a quadriplegic patient who can't move any part of his body except his mouth.

Attach a metal whistle to a piece of oxygen tubing and tape the tubing to the patient's face, near his mouth. He can then grasp the tubing with his tongue and blow into it to signal you. As a bonus, blowing the whistle also exercises his lungs.

—MARSHA URBEN, RN

LAST THINGS FIRST

If you're teaching newly diagnosed insulin-dependent diabetic patients about their disease, begin by carefully assessing each patient's needs. Then decide which patients are ready for self-injection practice sessions, and which are better started off with films and literature.

This way, patients who are apprehensive about the "real thing" can get it over with quickly. After learning how to inject themselves successfully, they're much more receptive to the other information that remains to be taught.

—NANCY RUFLI STEPTER, RN

QUICK REFERENCE GUIDE

COMMON POISONOUS PLANTS

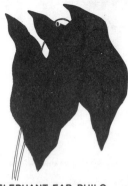

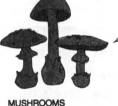

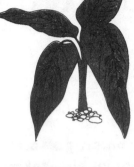

ELEPHANT EAR PHILO-DENDRON
Sx: burning throat and GI distress
Rx: gastric lavage or emesis; antihistamines and lime juice; symptomatic treatment

RHUBARB
Sx: GI and respiratory distress, internal bleeding, coma
Rx: gastric lavage or emesis with lime water; calcium gluconate and force fluids

DIEFFENBACHIA
Sx: burning throat, edema, GI distress
Rx: gastric lavage or emesis; antihistamines and lime juice; symptomatic treatment

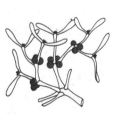

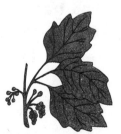

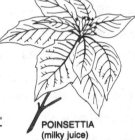

MISTLETOE
Sx: GI distress and slow pulse
Rx: gastric lavage or emesis; cardiac drugs, potassium, and sodium

MUSHROOMS
Sx: GI, respiratory, CNS, parasympathomimetic effects
Rx: lavage with potassium permanganate; saline catharsis; atropine

POINSETTIA
(milky juice)
Sx: inflammation and blisters
Rx: none; condition will disappear after several days

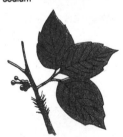

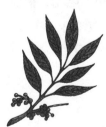

POISON IVY, POISON SUMAC, POISON OAK (sap)
Sx: allergic skin reactions; if ingested, GI distress, liver and kidney damage
Rx: if ingested: demulcents, morphine, fluids; high-protein low-fat diet. For skin reactions: antihistamine, topical antipyretics.

Poisonous parts of the plant are shaded. If the poisonous part can't be shown, it appears in parentheses after the plant's name.

From the NURSE'S REFERENCE LIBRARY volume *Diseases*, published by Intermed Communications, Inc., Springhouse, Pa. 1981.

SPECIAL AIDS FOR PREVENTING AND TREATING DECUBITUS ULCERS

Pressure relief aids:
- *Gel flotation pads* disperse pressure over a greater skin surface area, and are relatively convenient and adaptable for home and wheelchair use.
- *Water mattress* distributes body weight equally but is heavy and awkward; "mini" water beds (partially filled rubber gloves or plastic bags) may be used for small areas, such as heels and feet.
- *Alternating pressure mattress* contains tubelike sections, running lengthwise, that deflate and reinflate, changing areas of pressure; however, this mattress is noisy and its effectiveness remains unproven. It should be used with a single untucked sheet, since multiple layers of linen decrease its effectiveness. Make sure all connections are secure and that there are no kinks in the air hoses.
- *Egg crate mattress* minimizes area of skin pressure with its alternating areas of depression and elevation: soft, elevated foam areas cushion skin; depressed areas relieve pressure. This mattress should be used with a single, loosely tucked sheet and is adaptable for home and wheelchair use. If the patient is incontinent, cover mattress with the provided plastic sleeve.
- *Sheepskin* is soft, dry, absorbent, and easy to clean. It should be in direct contact with the patient's skin. Sheepskin is available in sizes to fit elbows and heels and is easily adaptable to home use.

- *Turning bed* is available in various makes and models (Stryker or Foster frame, Circ-Olectric bed, Roto-Rest). A turning bed is ineffective without adjuvant therapy. It also limits free movement, and is expensive and impractical for general use.

Topical agents:
- Gentle soap
- Zinc oxide cream
- Absorbable gelatin sponge
- Granulated sugar (mechanical irritant to enhance granulation)
- Dextranomer (inert, absorbing beads)
- Karaya gum patches
- Polyethylene dressings
- Topical antibiotics (*only* when infection is confirmed by culture and sensitivity tests)
- Silver sulfadiazine cream (antimicrobial agent)
- Oxychlorosene calcium (antiseptic used for irrigations and wet-to-dry packs, in 0.4% solution)
- Povidone-iodine packs (remain in place until dry)

Avoid the following skin-damaging agents:
- Harsh alkali soaps
- Alcohol-based products (witch hazel and astringents), which can cause vasoconstriction
- Tincture of benzoin (may cause painful erosions)
- Hexachlorophene (may irritate the central nervous system).

From the NURSE'S REFERENCE LIBRARY volume *Diseases*, published by Intermed Communications, Inc., Springhouse, Pa. 1981.

129

	atropine	butorphanol	chlorpromazine	codeine	diazepam	glycopyrrolate	hydromorphone
atropine		Y	P		N	Y	
butorphanol	Y		P		N	Y	
chlorpromazine	P	P			N	Y	
codeine					N	Y	
diazepam	N	N	N	N		N	N
glycopyrrolate	Y	Y	Y	Y	N		Y
hydromorphone					N	Y	
hydroxyzine	P	Y	P	P	N	Y	
meperidine	P		P		N	Y	
morphine	P		P		N	Y	
nalbuphine	Y				N	Y	
pentobarbital	P	N	N	N	N	N	
phenobarbital		N	N		N		
promethazine	P	Y	P		N	Y	
scopolamine	P	Y	P		N	Y	
secobarbital		N	N		N	N	
sodium bicarbonate	N		N	N	N	N	N
thiopental		N	N		N	N	N

KEY   Y = compatible   N = not compatible
P = provisionally compatible; use within 15 minutes of preparation

hydroxyzine	meperidine	morphine	nalbuphine	pentobarbital	phenobarbital	promethazine	scopolamine	secobarbital	sodium bicarbonate	thiopental
P	P	P	Y	P		P	P		N	
Y				N	N	Y	Y	N		N
P	P	P		N	N	P	P	N	N	N
P				N					N	
N	N	N	N	N	N	N	N	N	N	N
Y	Y	Y	Y	N		Y	Y	N	N	N
									N	N
■	P	P	Y	N	N	P	P		N	
P	■	N		N	N	P	P		N	N
P	N	■		?	N	?	P		N	N
Y			■			N	Y			
N	N	?		■		N	P		?	P
N	N	N			■	N				Y
P	P	?	N	N	N	■	P			N
P	P	P	Y	P		P	■	N	N	Y
							N	■		
N	N	N		?			N		■	N
	N	N		P	Y	N	Y		N	■

? = conflicting reports on compatibility; mixing not recommended
(A blank space indicates no available data on compatibility.)

From the *Nursing82 Drug Handbook*, published by Intermed Communications, Inc., Springhouse Pa. 1982.

COMMON ARTERIAL AND VENOUS PUNCTURE SITES

ARTERIES USED FOR ARTERIAL PUNCTURE

VEINS USED FOR VENIPUNCTURE

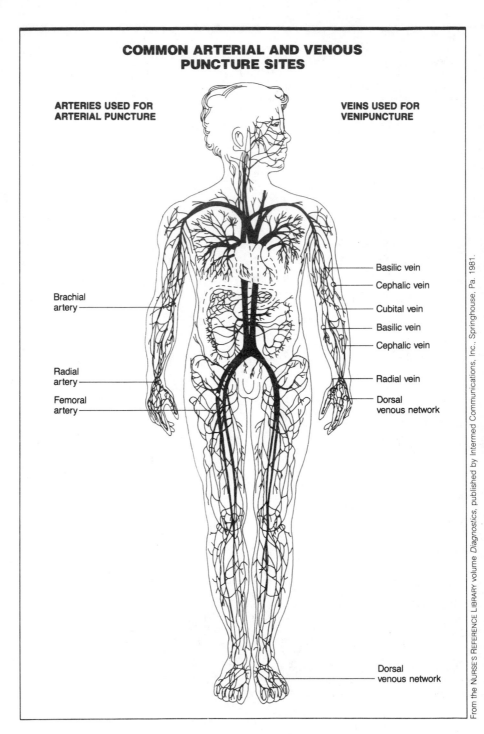

Basilic vein

Cephalic vein

Brachial artery

Cubital vein

Basilic vein

Cephalic vein

Radial artery

Radial vein

Femoral artery

Dorsal venous network

Dorsal venous network

From the NURSE'S REFERENCE LIBRARY volume *Diagnostics*, published by Intermed Communications, Inc., Springhouse, Pa. 1981.

GUIDE TO COLLECTING A VENOUS SAMPLE

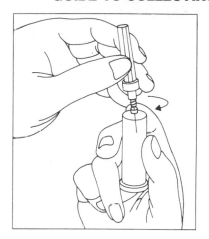

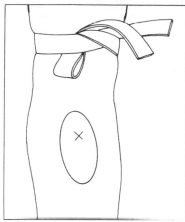

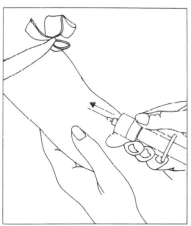

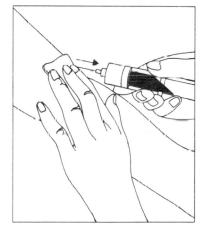

- Select a venipuncture site, usually the antecubital fossa.

- Using a circular motion, cleanse the area first with povidone-iodine solution and then alcohol.

- Screw the Vacutainer needle into the sleeve (top left).

- Apply a soft rubber tourniquet above the venipuncture site (top right).

- Remove the needle cover. With the bevel facing up, insert the needle into the patient's vein at a 15° angle (bottom left). When a drop of blood appears just inside the needle holder, gently push the Vacutainer tube into the needle sleeve, so the blood enters the tube. Try to keep the needle still to prevent it from perforating the patient's vein.

- When the tube is filled, remove the tourniquet, and pull the Vacutainer tube off the needle end. Withdraw the needle, using a dry sponge to apply direct pressure to the puncture site (bottom right). After 2 or 3 minutes, remove the sponge, and cover the site with an adhesive bandage.

From the NURSE'S REFERENCE LIBRARY volume *Diagnostics*, published by Intermec Communications, Inc., Springhouse, Pa 1981

133

QUICK TEST OF ARTERIAL FUNCTION

Before inserting an arterial line in one of your patient's radial arteries, assess the blood supply to your patient's hand. If the radial artery is blocked by a blood clot—a frequent complication of arterial lines—the ulnar artery alone must supply blood to the hand. The Allen's test is a simple, reliable procedure that quickly assesses arterial function.

Just follow these steps:

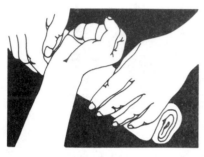

1 First, have the patient rest his arm on the bedside table. Support his wrist with a rolled towel. Ask him to clench his fist.

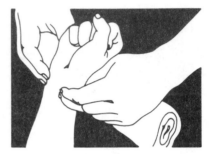

2 Now, use your index and middle fingers to exert pressure over both the radial and the ulnar arteries.

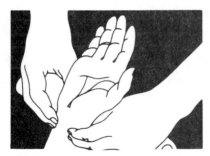

3 Without removing your fingers, ask the patient to unclench his fist. You'll notice his palm is blanched because you've impaired the normal blood flow with your fingers.
Nursing tip: Suppose your patient's unconscious or unable to clench his fist for some other reason. You can encourage his palm to blanch by occluding both arteries, elevating his hand, and massaging his palm.

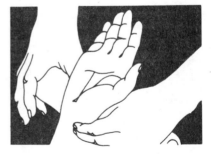

4 Release the pressure on the ulnar artery, and ask the patient to open his hand. If the ulnar artery's functioning well, his palm will turn pink in about 5 seconds, even though the radial artery's still occluded. But if blood return is slow and his fingers begin to contract, blood supply from the radial artery may not be adequate. In that case, try the Allen's test on his other wrist; you may get better results. *Note:* Slow blood return doesn't always indicate arterial occlusion. It may indicate poor cardiac output or poor capillary refill, resulting from shock.

From the NURSE'S REFERENCE LIBRARY volume *Diagnostics*, published by Intermed Communications, Inc., Springhouse, Pa. 1981.

IMPORTANT DEFINITIONS FOR UNDERSTANDING BLOOD GASES AND ELECTROLYTES

Partial pressure	A measure of the force that a gas exerts on the fluid in which it is dissolved
Pao$_2$	Partial pressure of oxygen in arterial blood
Paco$_2$	Partial pressure of carbon dioxide in arterial blood
pH	A measure of acid-base balance or the concentration of free hydrogen ions in the blood
O$_2$CT	Oxygen content, or the volume of oxygen combined with hemoglobin in arterial blood
O$_2$ Sat	Oxygen saturation, a measure of the percentage of oxygen combined with hemoglobin to the total amount of oxygen with which hemoglobin could combine
Electrolytes	Substances that dissociate into ions when fused or in solution, and thus conduct electricity
Cations	Positively charged ions
Anions	Negatively charged ions
Acidosis	Metabolic or respiratory changes that result in a loss of base or accumulation of acid
Alkalosis	Metabolic or respiratory changes that result in a loss of acid or accumulation of base

From the NURSE'S REFERENCE LIBRARY volume *Diagnostics*, published by Intermed Communications, Inc., Springhouse, Pa. 1981.

135

LABORATORY TEST VALUES

A

Acid phosphatase, serum
0 to 1.1 Bodansky units/ml
1 to 4 King-Armstrong units/ml
0.13 to 0.63 BLB units/ml

ACTH, plasma
< 120 pg/ml

ACTH, rapid test, plasma
Cortisol rises 7 to 18 mcg/dl above
baseline, 60 minutes after injection

Activated partial thromboplastin time
25 to 36 seconds

Albumin, peritoneal fluid
50% to 70% of total protein

Albumin, serum
3.3 to 4.5 g/dl

Aldosterone, serum
1 to 21 ng/dl (standing)

Aldosterone, urine
2 to 16 mcg/24 hours

Alkaline phosphatase, peritoneal fluid
Men: > age 18, 90 to 239 units/liter
Women: < age 45, 76 to 196 units/
liter; > age 45, 87 to 250 units/liter

Alkaline phosphatase, serum
1.5 to 4 Bodansky units/dl
4 to 13.5 King-Armstrong units/dl
Chemical inhibition method: Men,
90 to 239 units/dl; Women; < age
45, 76 to 196 units/liter;
Women > age 45, 87 to 250
units/liter

Alpha-fetoprotein, amniotic fluid
≤ 18.5 mcg/ml at 13 or 14 weeks

Alpha-fetoprotein, serum
Nonpregnant females: < 30 ng/ml

Amino acids, urine
50 to 200 mg/24 hours

Ammonia, peritoneal fluid
< 50 mcg/dl

Ammonia, plasma
< 50 mcg/dl

Amniotic fluid
Meconium: Absent
Lecithin/sphingomyelin ratio: > 2
Phosphatidiglycerol: Present
Bacteria: Absent

Amylase, peritoneal fluid
138 to 404 amylase units/liter

Amylase, serum
60 to 180 Somogyi units/dl

Amylase, urine
10 to 80 amylase units/hour

Antibody screening, serum
Negative

Anti–deoxyribonucleic acid antibodies, serum
< 1 mcg DNA bound/ml

Antidiuretic hormone, serum
1 to 5 pg/ml

Antiglobulin test, direct
Negative

Antimitochondrial antibodies, serum
Negative at 1:5 dilution

Antinuclear antibodies, serum
Negative at ≤ 1:32 titer

Anti–smooth-muscle antibodies, serum
Normal titer < 1:20

Antistreptolysin-O, serum
< 85 Todd units/ml

Antithyroid antibodies, serum
Normal titer < 1:100

Arterial blood gases
Pao_2:   75 to 100 mmHg
$Paco_2$: 35 to 45 mmHg
pH: 7.35 to 7.42
O_2CT: 15% to 23%
O_2 *Sat*: 94% to 100%
HCO_3^-: 22 to 26 mEq/liter

Arylsulfatase A, urine
Men: 1.4 to 19.3 units/liter
Women: 1.4 to 11 units/liter

Aspergillosis antibody, serum
Normal titer < 1:8

B

B-lymphocyte count
270 to 640/mm³

Bence Jones protein, urine
Negative

Bilirubin, amniotic fluid
Absent at term

Bilirubin, serum

Adult: Direct, < 0.5 mg/dl; indirect, ≤ 1.1 mg/dl
Neonate: Total, 1 to 12 mg/dl

Bilirubin, urine
Negative

Blastomycosis antibody, serum
Normal titer < 1:8

Bleeding time
Template: 2 to 8 minutes
Ivy: 1 to 7 minutes
Duke: 1 to 3 minutes

Blood urea nitrogen
8 to 20 mg/dl

C

C-reactive protein, serum
Negative

Calcitonin, plasma
Baseline: Males, ≤ 0.155 ng/ml; females, ≤ 0.105 ng/ml
Calcium infusion: Males, 0.265 ng/ml; females, 0.120 ng/ml
Pentagastrin infusion: Males, 0.210 ng/ml; females, 0.105 ng/ml

Calcium, serum
4.5 to 5.5 mEq/liter
Atomic absorption: 8.9 to 10.1 mg/dl

Calcium, urine
Males: < 275 mg/24 hours
Females: < 250 mg/24 hours

Calculi, urine
None

Capillary fragility

Petechiae:		Score:	
0 to 10		1 +	
10 to 20		2 +	
20 to 50		3 +	
50		4 +	

Carbon dioxide, total, blood
22 to 34 mEq/liter

Carcinoembryonic antigen, serum
< 5 ng/ml

Carotene, serum
48 to 200 mcg/dl

Catecholamines, plasma
Supine: Epinephrine, 0 to 110 pg/ml; norepinephrine, 70 to 750 pg/ml; dopamine, 0 to 30 pg/ml
Standing: Epinephrine, 0 to 140 pg/ml; norepinephrine, 200 to 1,700 pg/ml; and dopamine, 0 to 30 pg/ml

Catecholamines, urine
24-hour specimen: 0 to 135 mcg
Random specimen: 0 to 18 mcg/dl

Catheterization, pulmonary artery
Right atrial: 1 to 6 mmHg

Systolic right ventricular: 20 to 30 mmHg
End diastolic right ventricular: < 5 mmHg
Systolic PAP: 20 to 30 mmHg
Diastolic PAP: approximately 10 mmHg
Mean PAP: < 20 mmHg
PAWP: 6 to 12 mmHg
Left atrial: approximately 10 mmHg

Cerebrospinal fluid
Pressure: 50 to 180 mm water
Appearance: Clear, colorless
Gram's stain: No organisms

Ceruloplasmin, serum
22.9 to 43.1 mg/dl

Chloride, cerebrospinal fluid
118 to 130 mEq/liter

Chloride, serum
100 to 108 mEq/liter

Chloride, sweat
10 to 35 mEq/liter

Chloride, urine
110 to 250 mEq/24 hours

Cholesterol, total, serum
120 to 330 mg/dl

Cholinesterase (pseudocholinesterase)
8 to 18 units/ml

Chorionic gonadotropin, serum
< 3 mIU/ml

Chorionic gonadotropin, urine
Pregnant females: First trimester, ≤ 500,000 IU/24 hours; second trimester, 10,000 to 25,000 IU/24 hours; third trimester, 5,000 to 15,000 IU/24 hours

Clot retraction
50%

Coccidioidomycosis antibody, serum
Normal titer < 1:2

Cold agglutinins, serum
Normal titer < 1:16

Complement, serum
Total: 41 to 90 hemolytic units
CI esterase inhibitor: 16 to 33 mg/dl
C3: Males, 88 to 252 mg/dl; females, 88 to 206 mg/dl
C4: Males, 12 to 72 mg/dl; females, 13 to 75 mg/dl

Complement, synovial fluid
10 mg protein/dl: 3.7 to 33.7 units/ml
20 mg protein/dl: 7.7 to 37.7 units/ml

Copper, urine
15 to 60 mcg/24 hours

Copper reduction test, urine

From the NURSE'S REFERENCE LIBRARY volume *Diagnostics*, published by Intermed Communications, Inc., Springhouse, Pa. 1981.

Negative
Coproporphyrin, urine
Men: 0 to 96 mcg/24 hours
Women: 1 to 57 mcg/24 hours
Cortisol, plasma
Morning: 7 to 28 mcg/dl
Afternoon: 2 to 18 mcg/dl
Cortisol, free, urine
24 to 108 mcg/24 hours
Creatine phosphokinase
Total: Men, 23 to 99 units/liter; women,
15 to 57 units/liter
CPK-BB: None
CPK-MB: 0 to 7 IU/liter
CPK-MM: 5 to 70 IU/liter
Creatine, serum
Males: 0.2 to 0.6 mg/dl
Females: 0.6 to 1 mg/dl
Creatinine, amniotic fluid
> 2 mg/100 ml in mature fetus
Creatinine clearance
Men (age 20): 90 ml/minute/1.73 m²
Women (age 20): 84 ml/minute/1.73
m²
Creatinine, serum
Males: 0.8 to 1.2 mg/dl
Females: 0.6 to 0.9 mg/dl
Creatinine, urine
Men: 1 to 1.9 g/24 hours
Women: 0.8 to 1.7 g/24 hours
Cryoglobulins, serum
Negative
Cryptococcosis antigen, serum
Negative
Cyclic adenosine monophosphate, urine
Parathyroid hormone infusion: 3.6 to
4 μmoles increase

D
Delta-aminolevulinic acid, urine
1.5 to 7.5 mg/dl/24 hours
D-xylose absorption
Blood: Children, 730 mg/dl in 1 hour;
adults, 25 to 40 mg/dl in 2 hours
Urine: Children, 16 to 33% excreted in
5 hours; adults, > 3.5 g excreted in
5 hours

E
Erythrocyte sedimentation rate
Males: 0 to 10 mm/hour
Females: 0 to 20 mm/hour
Esophageal acidity
pH > 5.0
Estriol, amniotic fluid

16 to 20 weeks: 25.7 ng/ml
Term: < 1,000 ng/ml
Estrogens, serum
Menstruating females: day 1 to 10,
24 to 68 pg/ml; day 11 to 20, 50 to
186 pg/ml; day 21 to 30, 73 to 149
pg/ml
Males: 12 to 34 pg/ml
Estrogens, total urine
Menstruating females: follicular phase,
5 to 25 mcg/24 hours; ovulatory
phase, 24 to 100 mcg/24 hours;
luteal phase, 12 to 80 mcg/24 hours
Postmenopausal females: < 10 mcg/
24 hours
Males: 4 to 25 mcg/24 hours
Euglobulin lysis time
≥ 2 hours

F
Factor II assay
225 to 290 units/ml
Factor V assay
50% to 150% of control
Factor VII assay
65% to 135% of control
Factor VIII assay
55% to 145% of control
Factor IX assay
60% to 140% of control
Factor X assay
45% to 155% of control
Factor XI assay
65% to 135% of control
Factor XII assay
50% to 150% of control
Febrile agglutination, serum
Salmonella *antibody:* < 1:80
Brucellosis *antibody:* < 1:80
Tularemia *antibody:* < 1:40
Rickettsial *antibody:* < 1:40
Ferritin, serum
Men: 20 to 300 ng/ml
Women: 20 to 120 ng/ml
Fibrin split products
Screening assay: < 10 mcg/ml
Quantitative assay: < 3 mcg/ml
Fibrinogen, peritoneal fluid
0.3% to 4.5% of total protein
Fibrinogen, plasma
195 to 365 mg/dl
Fibrinogen, pleural fluid
Transudate: Absent
Exudate: Present
Fibrinogen, synovial fluid

None
Fluorescent treponemal absorption, serum
Negative
Folic acid, serum
2 to 14 ng/ml
Follicle-stimulating hormone, serum
Menstruating females: Follicular phase, 5 to 20 mIU/ml; ovulatory phase, 15 to 30 mIU/ml; luteal phase, 5 to 15 mIU//ml
Menopausal women: 5 to 100 mIU/ml
Males: 5 to 20 mIU/ml
Free fatty acids, plasma
0.3 to 1.0 mEq/liter
Free thyroxine, serum
0.8 to 3.3 ng/dl
Free triiodothyronine
0.2 to 0.6 ng/dl

G

Gamma glutamyl transferase
Males: 6 to 37 units/liter
Females: < age 45, 5 to 27 units/liter; > age 45, 6 to 37 units/liter
Gastric acid stimulation
Males: 18 to 28 mEq/hour
Females: 11 to 21 mEq/hour
Gastric secretion, basal
Males: 1 to 5 mEq/hour
Females: 0.2 to 3.8 mEq/hour
Gastrin, serum
< 300 pg/ml
Globulin, peritoneal fluid
30% to 45% of total protein
Globulin, serum
$Alpha_1$: 0.1 to 0.4 g/dl
$Alpha_2$: 0.5 to 1 g/dl
Beta: 0.7 to 1.2 g/dl
Gamma: 0.5 to 1.6 g/dl
Glucose, amniotic fluid
< 45 mg/100 ml
Glucose, cerebrospinal fluid
50 to 80 mg/100 ml
Glucose, fasting, plasma
70 to 100 mg/dl
Glucose, peritoneal fluid
70 to 100 mg/dl
Glucose, plasma, oral tolerance
Peak at 160 to 180 mg/dl, 30 to 60 minutes after challenge dose
Glucose, plasma, 2-hour postprandial
< 145 mg/dl
Glucose, synovial fluid

70 to 100 mg/dl
Glucose, urine
Negative
Growth hormone, serum
Men: 0 to 5 ng/ml
Women: 0 to 10 ng/ml
Growth hormone stimulation
Men: Increases to ≥ 10 ng/ml
Women: Increases to ≥ 15 ng/ml
Growth hormone suppression
0 to 3 ng/ml after 30 minutes to 2 hours

H

Haptoglobin, serum
38 to 270 mg/dl
Heinz bodies
Negative
Hematocrit
Men: 42% to 54%
Women: 38% to 46%
Hemoglobin electrophoresis
Hgb A: 95%
$Hgb A_2$: 2% to 3%
Hgb F: > 1%
Hemoglobin, glycosylated
$Hgb A_{1a}$: 1.6% of total RBC Hgb
$Hgb A_{1b}$: 0.8% of total RBC Hgb
$Hgb A_{1c}$: 4% of total RBC Hgb
Total glycosylated Hgb: 5.5% to 9%
Hemoglobin, total
Men: 14 to 18 g/dl
Women: 12 to 16 g/dl
Hemoglobin, urine
Negative
Hemoglobins, unstable
Heat stability: Negative
Isopropanol: Stable
Hemosiderin, urine
Negative
Hepatitis-B surface antigen, serum
Negative
Heterophil agglutination, serum
Normal titer < 1:56
Hexosaminidase A and B, serum
Total: 5 to 12.9 units/liter (Hex-A is 55% to 76% of total)
Histoplasmosis antibody, serum
Normal titer: < 1:8
Homovanillic acid, urine
< 8 mg/24 hours
Hydroxybutyric dehydrogenase
Serum HBD: 114 to 290 units/ml
LDH/HBD ratio: 1.2 to 1.6:1
17-Hydroxycorticosteroids, urine

Men: 4.5 to 12 mg/24 hours
Women: 2.5 to 10 mg/24 hours
5-Hydroxyindoleacetic acid, urine
< 6 mg/24 hours

I

Immune complex assays, serum
Negative
Immunoglobulins, serum
IgG: 6.4 to 14.3 mg/ml
IgA: 0.3 to 3 mg/ml
IgM: 0.2 to 1.4 mg/ml
Insulin, serum
0 to 25 μU/ml
Inulin clearance, urine
≥ *Age 21:* 90 to 130 ml/minute
Iron, serum
Men: 70 to 150 mcg/dl
Women: 80 to 150 mcg/dl
Iron, total binding capacity, serum
Men: 300 to 400 mcg/dl (20% to 50% saturation)
Women: 300 to 450 mcg/dl (20% to 50% saturation)
Isocitrate dehydrogenase
1.2 to 7 units/liter

J, K

17-Ketogenic steroids, urine
Men: 4 to 14 mg/24 hours
Women: 2 to 12 mg/24 hours
Ketones, urine
Negative
17-Ketosteroids, urine
Men: 6 to 21 mg/24 hours
Women: 4 to 17 mg/24 hours

L

Lactic acid, blood
0.93 to 1.65 mEq/liter
Lactic dehydrogenase
Total: 48 to 115 IU/liter
LDH_1: 18.1% to 29%
LDH_2: 29.4% to 37.5%
LDH_3: 18.8% to 26%
LDH_4: 9.2% to 16.5%
LDH_5: 5.3% to 13.4%
Leucine aminopeptidase
< 50 units/liter
Lipase
32 to 80 units/liter
Lipids, amniotic fluid
> 20% of lipid-coated cells stain orange
Lipids, fecal

< 20% of excreted solids; < 7 g/24 hours
Lipoproteins, serum
HDL-cholesterol: 29 to 77 mg/dl
LDL-cholesterol: 62 to 185 mg/dl
Long-acting thyroid stimulator, serum
Negative
Lupus erythematosus cell preparation
Negative
Lupus erythematosus cells, synovial fluid
None
Luteinizing hormone, plasma
Menstruating females: Follicular phase, 5 to 15 mIU/ml; ovulatory phase, 30 to 60 mIU/ml; luteal phase, 5 to 15 mIU/ml
Postmenopausal females: 50 to 100 mIU/ml
Men: 5 to 20 mIU/ml
Lymphocyte transformation
60% to 90% lymphocytes respond to nonspecific antigens
Lysozyme, urine
< 3 mg/24 hours

M

Magnesium, serum
1.5 to 2.5 mEq/liter
Atomic absorption: 1.7 to 2.1 mg/dl
Magnesium, urine
< 150 mg/24 hours
Manganese, serum
0.4 to 0.85 ng/ml
Melanin, urine
Negative
Myoglobin, urine
Negative

N

5′ - Nucleotidase
2 to 17 units/liter

O

Occult blood, fecal
< 2.5 ml/24 hours
Ornithine carbamoyltransferase, serum
0 to 500 Sigma units/ml
Oxalate, urine
≤ 40 mg/24 hours

P

Para-aminohippuric acid excretion, urine

Age 20: 400 to 700 ml/minute (17 ml/minute decrease each decade after age 20)

Parathyroid hormone, serum
20 to 70 μlEq/ml

Pericardial fluid
Amount: 10 to 50 ml
Appearance: Clear, straw-colored
Pathogens: None
Blood: None
Cytology: No malignant cells
White blood cell count: < 1,000/mm³
Glucose: approximately whole blood level

Peritoneal fluid
Amount: < 50 ml
Appearance: Clear, straw-colored
Cytology: No malignant cells
Fungi: None
Bacteria: None

Phenylalanine, serum, screening
Negative: < 2 mg/dl

Phenolsulfonphthalein excretion, urine
15 minutes: 25% of dose excreted
30 minutes: 50% to 60% of dose excreted
1 hour: 60% to 79% of dose excreted
2 hours: 70% to 80% of dose excreted

Phosphates, serum
1.8 to 2.6 mEq/liter
Atomic absorption: 2.5 to 4.5 mg/dl

Phosphates, urine
< 1,000 mg/24 hours

Phosphate, tubular reabsorption, urine and plasma
80% reabsorption

Phospholipids, plasma
180 to 320 mg/dl

Phytanic acid, serum
< 0.3% of blood lipids

Placental lactogen, serum
Pregnant females: 5 to 27 weeks, < 4.6 mcg/ml; 28 to 31 weeks, 2.4 to 6.1 mcg/ml; 32 to 35 weeks, 3.7 to 7.7 mcg/ml; 36 weeks to term, 5 to 8.6 mcg/ml
Nonpregnant females: < 0.5 mcg/ml
Males: < 0.5 mcg/ml

Plasma renin activity
Sodium-depleted, peripheral vein (upright position): Ages 20 to 39, 2.9 to 24 ng/ml/hour (mean–10.8 ng/ml/hour); age 40 and over, 2.9 to 10.8 ng/ml/hour (mean–5.9 ng/ml/hour)
Sodium-replete, peripheral vein (upright position): Ages 20 to 39, 0.1 to 4.3 ng/ml/hour (mean–1.9 ng/ml/hour); age 40 and over, 0.1 to 3 ng/ml/hour (mean–1 ng/ml/hour)
Renal venous renin ratio: < 1.5:1

Platelet aggregation
3 to 5 minutes

Platelet count
130,000 to 370,000/mm³

Platelet survival
50% tagged platelets disappear within 84 to 116 hours
100% disappear within 8 to 10 days

Pleural fluid
Appearance: Clear (transudate); cloudy, turbulent (exudate)
Specific gravity: < 1.016 (transudate); > 1.016 (exudate)

Porphobilinogen, urine
≤ 1.5 mg/24 hours

Potassium, serum
3.8 to 5.5 mEq/liter

Pregnanediol, urine
Males: 1.5 mg/24 hours
Females: 0.5 to 1.5 mg/24 hours
Postmenopausal females: 0.2 to 1 mg/24 hours

Pregnanetriol, urine
< 3.5 mg/24 hours

Progesterone, plasma
Menstrual cycle: Follicular phase, < 150 ng/dl; luteal phase, 300 ng/dl; midluteal phase, 2,000 ng/dl
Pregnancy: First trimester, 1,500 to 5,000 ng/dl; second and third trimesters, 8,000 to 20,000 ng/dl

Prolactin, serum
0 to 23 ng/dl

Protein, cerebrospinal fluid
15 to 45 mg/dl

Protein, pleural fluid
Transudate: < 3 g/dl
Exudate: > 3 g/dl

Protein, total, peritoneal fluid
0.3 to 4.1 g/dl

Protein, total, serum
6.6 to 7.9 g/dl
Albumin fraction: 3.3 to 4.5 g/dl
Globulin levels: Alpha₁–globulin, 0.1 to 0.4 g/dl; alpha₂–globulin, 0.5 to 1 g/dl; beta globulin, 0.7 to 1.2 g/dl; gamma globulin, 0.5 to 1.6 g/dl

Protein, total, synovial fluid

10.7 to 21.3 mg/dl

Protein, urine
≤ 150 mg/24 hours

Prothrombin consumption time
20 seconds

Prothrombin time
Males: 9.6 to 11.8 seconds
Females: 9.5 to 11.3 seconds

Pyruvate kinase
Ultraviolet: 2 to 8.8 units/g hemoglobin
Low substrate assay: 0.9 to 3.9 units/g
hemoglobin

Pyruvic acid, blood
0.08 to 0.16 mEq/liter

R

Radioallergosorbent test
Negative: < 150% of control

Red blood cell count
Men: 4.5 to 6.2 million/µl venous blood
Women: 4.2 to 5.4 million/µl venous
blood

Red blood cells, cerebrospinal fluid
None

Red blood cells, peritoneal fluid
None

Red blood cells, pleural fluid
. *Transudate:* Few
Exudate: Variable

Red blood cells, urine
0 to 3 per high-power field

Red cell indices
MCH: 26 to 32 pg/red cell
MCHC: 30% to 36%
MCV: 84 to 99 µ³/red cell

Reticulocyte count
0.5% to 2% of total RBC count

Rheumatoid factor, serum
Negative

Rubella antibodies, serum
Titer of 1:8 or less indicates little or no
immunity

S

Semen
Volume: 1.5 to 5 ml
pH: 7.3 to 7.7
Liquefaction: 30 minutes
Sperm count: 60 to 150 million/ml
Cervical mucus: ≥ 5 motile sperm per
high-power field
Spinnbarkeit: 4" (10 cm)

Serum glutamic-oxaloacetic
transaminase
8 to 20 units/liter

Serum glutamic-pyruvic transaminase
Men: 10 to 32 units/liter
Women: 9 to 24 units/liter

Sickle cell test
Negative

Sodium, serum
135 to 145 mEq/liter

Sodium, sweat
10 to 30 mEq/liter

Sodium, urine
30 to 280 mEq/24 hours

Sodium chloride, urine
5 to 20 g/24 hours

Sporotrichosis antibody, serum
Normal titers < 1:40

Sulfobromophthalein excretion
90% complete in 45 minutes

Synovial fluid
Color: Colorless to pale yellow
Clarity: Clear
Quantity (in knee): 0.3 to 3.5 ml
Viscosity: 5.7 to 1,160
pH: 7.2 to 7.4
Mucin clot: Good
Bacteria: None
Formed elements: None
Pao$_2$: 40 to 60 mmHg
Paco$_2$: 40 to 60 mmHg

T

T-lymphocyte count
1,400 to 2,700/mm³

T$_3$ resin uptake
25% to 35% of T$_3$* binds resin

Testosterone, plasma or serum
Men: 30 to 1,200 ng/dl
Women: 30 to 95 ng/dl

Thrombin time, plasma
10 to 15 seconds

Thyroid-stimulating hormone, serum
0 to 15 µIU/ml

Thyroxine, total, serum
5 to 13.5 mcg/dl

Thyroxine-binding globulin, serum
Electrophoresis: From 10 to 26 mcg T$_4$
(binding capacity)/dl to 16 to 24 mcg
T$_4$ (binding capacity)/dl (depending
on the laboratory)
Radioimmunoassay: 1.3 to 2 ng/dl

Tolbutamide tolerance
Plasma glucose drops to one half
fasting level for 30 minutes, recovers
in 1½ to 3 hours

Transferrin, serum
250 to 390 mcg/dl

Triglycerides, serum
  Ages 0 to 29: 10 to 140 mg/dl
  Ages 30 to 39: 10 to 150 mg/dl
  Ages 40 to 49: 10 to 160 mg/dl
  Ages 50 to 59: 10 to 190 mg/dl
Triiodothyronine, serum
  90 to 230 ng/dl

U

Urea, urine
  Maximal clearance: 64 to 99 ml/minute
Uric acid, serum
  Men: 4.3 to 8 mg/dl
  Women: 2.3 to 6 mg/dl
Uric acid, synovial fluid
  Men: 2 to 8 mg/dl
  Women: 2 to 6 mg/dl
Uric acid, urine
  250 to 750 mg/24 hours
Urinalysis, routine
  Color: Straw
  Odor: Slightly aromatic
  Appearance: Clear
  Specific gravity: 1.025 to 1.030
  pH: 4.5 to 8.0
  Sugars: None
  Epithelial cells: Few
  Casts: None, except occasional
    hyaline casts
  Crystals: Present
  Yeast cells: None
Urine concentration
  Specific gravity: 1.025 to 1.032
  Osmolality: > 800 mOsm/kg water
Urine dilution
  Specific gravity: < 1.003
  Osmolality: < 100 mOsm/kg
  80% of water excreted in 4 hours
Urobilinogen, fecal
  50 to 300 mg/24 hours
Urobilinogen, urine
  Men: 0.3 to 2.1 Ehrlich units/2 hours
  Women: 0.1 to 1.1 Ehrlich units/
    2 hours
Uroporphyrin, urine
  Men: 0 to 42 mcg/24 hours
  Women: 1 to 22 mcg/24 hours

V

Vanillylmandelic acid, urine
  0.7 to 6.8 mg/24 hours
VDRL, cerebrospinal fluid
  Negative
VDRL, serum
  Negative

Vitamin A, serum
  125 to 150 IU/dl
Vitamin B$_1$, urine
  100 to 200 mcg/24 hours
Vitamin B$_2$, urine
  Males: 0.51 mg/24 hours
  Females: 0.39 mg/24 hours
Vitamin B$_6$, (tryptophan), urine
  < 50 mcg/24 hours
Vitamin B$_{12}$, serum
  200 to 1,100 pg/ml
Vitamin B$_{12}$ absorption, urine
  8% to 40% excreted/24 hours
Vitamin C, plasma
  0.2 to 2 mg/dl
Vitamin C, urine
  30 mg/24 hours
Vitamin D$_3$, serum
  10 to 55 ng/ml

W

White blood cell count, blood
  4,100 to 10,900/μl
White blood cell count, cerebrospinal fluid
  0 to 5/mm³
White blood cell count, peritoneal fluid
  < 300/μl
White blood cell count, pleural fluid
  Transudate: Few
  Exudate: Many (may be purulent)
White blood cell count, synovial fluid
  0 to 200/μl
White blood cell count, urine
  0 to 4 per high-power field
White blood cell differential, blood
  Neutrophils: 47.6% to 76.8%
  Lymphocytes: 16.2% to 43%
  Monocytes: 0.6% to 9.6%
  Eosinophils: 0.3% to 7%
  Basophils: 0.3% to 2%
White blood cell differential, synovial fluid
  Lymphocytes: 0 to 78/μl
  Monocytes: 0 to 71/μl
  Clasmatocytes: 0 to 26/μl
  Polymorphonuclears: 0 to 25/μl
  Other phagocytes: 0 to 21/μl
  Synovial lining cells: 0 to 12/μl
Whole blood clotting time
  5 to 15 minutes

Z

Zinc, serum
  0.75 to 1.4 mcg/ml

GUIDE TO COLOR-TOP COLLECTION TUBES

Red

Red-top tubes contain no additives. Draw volume may be 2 to 20 ml. These tubes are used for tests performed on serum samples.

ABO blood typing
Acid phosphatase
Alkaline phosphatase
Alpha-fetoprotein
Antibody screening test
Anti-DNA antibodies
Antimitochondrial antibodies
Antinuclear antibodies
Anti–smooth-muscle antibodies
Antistreptolysin-0 test
Antithyroid antibodies
Blood ethanol
Blood urea nitrogen
Carcinoembryonic antigen
Cholinesterase
Cold agglutinins
Complement assays
C-reactive protein
Creatine phosphokinase
Creatinine clearance
Crossmatching
Cryoglobulins
D-xylose absorption
Febrile agglutination tests
5'-nucleotidase
Fluorescent treponemal antibody absorption test
Free fatty acids
Fungal serology
Gamma glutamyl transferase
Growth hormone stimulation test (arginine test)
Growth hormone suppression test (glucose loading)
Hepatitis B surface antigen
Heterophil agglutination tests
Hydroxybutyric dehydrogenase
Immunoglobulins G, A, and M
Isocitrate dehydrogenase
Lactic dehydrogenase
LE cell preparation
Leucine aminopeptidase
Lipase
Lipoprotein-cholesterol fractionation

Ornithine carbamoyltransferase
Phospholipids
Phytanic acid
Plasma LH
Prolactin (lactogenic hormone, lactogen)
Prothrombin consumption time
Radioallergosorbent test
Rheumatoid factor
Rh typing
Rubella antibodies
Serum amylase
Serum antibiotics
Serum anticonvulsants
Serum antidiuretic hormone (vasopressin)
Serum antiglobulin
Serum bilirubin
Serum calcium
Serum ceruloplasmin
Serum chloride
Serum creatine
Serum creatinine
Serum estrogens
Serum ferritin
Serum folic acid
Serum FSH
Serum FT_4 and FT_3
Serum gastrin
Serum growth hormone/somatotropic hormone
Serum haptoglobin
Serum hexosaminidase A & B
Serum human chorionic gonadotropin
Serum human placental lactogen
Serum immune complex assays
Serum insulin
Serum iron and total iron-binding capacity
Serum long-acting thyroid stimulator
Serum magnesium
Serum parathyroid hormone (parathormone)
Serum phosphates
Serum potassium
Serum protein electrophoresis
Serum sodium
Serum testosterone
Serum TSH (thyrotropin)
Serum thyroxine
Serum thyroxine-binding globulin
Serum transferrin

Serum triiodothyronine
Serum uric acid
Serum vitamin A and carotene
Serum vitamin B_{12}
Serum vitamin D_3
SGOT
SGPT
Sulfobromophthalein excretion
T_3 resin uptake
Total cholesterol
Triglycerides
Tubular reabsorption of phosphate
Urea clearance
VDRL

Lavender

Lavender-top *tubes contain EDTA. Draw volume may be 2 to 10 ml. These tubes are used for tests performed on whole blood samples.*

Anti-DNA antibodies
Erythrocyte sedimentation rate
G-6-PD
Glycosylated hemoglobin
Heinz bodies
Hematocrit
Hemoglobin electrophoresis
Lipoprotein phenotyping
Plasma renin activity
Platelet count
Platelet survival
Pyruvate kinase
RBC count
Red cell indices
Reticulocyte count
Sickle cell test (hemoglobin S)
Total hemoglobin
Unstable hemoglobins
WBC count
White blood cell differential

Green (heparinized)

Green-top *tubes contain heparin (sodium, lithium, or ammonium). Draw volume may be 2 to 15 ml. These tubes are used for tests performed on plasma samples.*

Chromosomal analysis
Inulin clearance
Lymphocyte transformation tests
Osmotic fragility

Para-aminohippuric acid excretion
Plasma ACTH
Plasma ammonia
Plasma calcitonin (thryocalcitonin)
Plasma cortisol
Plasma progesterone
Plasma testosterone
Rapid ACTH (cosyntropin test)
T- and B-lymphocyte counts

Blue

Blue-top *tubes contain sodium citrate and citric acid. Draw volume may be 2.7 or 4.5 ml. These tubes are used for coagulation studies requiring plasma samples.*

Activated partial thromboplastin time
Euglobulin lysis time
Hemoglobin derivatives
One-stage assay: Extrinsic coagulation
    system
One-stage assay: Intrinsic coagulation
    system
Plasma fibrinogen
Plasma thrombin time
Platelet aggregation
Prothrombin time

Black

Black-top *tubes contain sodium oxalate. Draw volume may be 2.7 or 4.5 ml. These tubes are used for coagulation studies performed on plasma samples.*

Plasma vitamin C

Gray

Gray-top *tubes contain a glycolytic inhibitor (such as sodium fluoride, powdered oxalate, or glycolytic/microbial inhibitor). Draw volume may be 3 to 10 ml. These tubes are used most often for glucose determinations in serum or plasma samples.*

Anti-DNA antibodies
Fasting plasma glucose (fasting blood
    sugar)
Lactic acid and pyruvic acid
Oral glucose tolerance test
Tolbutamide tolerance test
Two-hour postprandial plasma glucose

From the *Nursing82 Drug Handbook*, published by Intermed Communications, Inc., Springhouse, Pa. 1982.

RECOMMENDED DAILY ALLOWANCE*

AGE GROUP	THIAMINE (VITAMIN B₁)	RIBOFLAVIN (VITAMIN B₂)	PYRIDOXINE PYRIDOXAL PYRIDOXAMINE (VITAMIN B₆)	CYANOCOBAL-AMIN (VITAMIN B₁₂)
Infants	0.4 mg	0.5 mg	0.4 mg	0.3 mcg
Children (1 to 10)	0.7 to 1.2 mg	0.8 to 1.2 mg	0.6 to 1.2 mg	1.0 to 2.0 mcg
Men (23 to 50)	1.4 mg	1.6 mg	2.0 mg	3 mcg
Women (23 to 50)	1.0 mg	1.2 mg	2.0 mg	3 mcg

*requirements per 1,000 kilocalories of dietary intake

From the NURSE'S REFERENCE LIBRARY volume *Diagnostics*, published by Intermed Communications, Inc., Springhouse, Pa. 1981.

SOURCES OF VITAMINS AND TRACE ELEMENTS

MICRONUTRIENT	FOOD SOURCES	DISORDERS
Thiamine (vitamin B₁)	Pork, liver, dried yeast, whole-grain cereals, enriched cereals, nuts, legumes, potatoes	Deficiency: beriberi
Riboflavin (vitamin B₂)	Milk, cheddar cheese, cottage cheese, liver, eggs, green leafy vegetables	Deficiency: ariboflavinosis
Pyridoxine (vitamin B₆)	Dried yeast, liver, whole-grain cereals, fish, legumes	Deficiency: pellagra
Cobalamin (vitamin B₁₂)	Liver, beef, pork, eggs, milk, milk products	Deficiency: pernicious anemia
Ascorbic acid (vitamin C)	Citrus fruits, tomatoes, potatoes, cabbage, green peppers	Deficiency: scurvy
Sodium	Table salt, beef, pork, sardines, cheese, milk, eggs	Toxicity: hypernatremia Deficiency: hyponatremia
Chloride	Table salt, seafood, milk, meat, eggs	Toxicity: hyperchloremia Deficiency: hypochloremia
Calcium	Milk, milk products, meat, fish, eggs, cereals, beans, fruit, vegetables	Toxicity: hypercalcemia Deficiency: hypocalcemia
Phosphorus	Milk, cheese, meat, poultry, fish, whole-grain cereals, nuts, legumes	Toxicity: hyperphosphatemia Deficiency: hypophosphatemia
Magnesium	Seafood, soybeans, nuts, cocoa, whole-grain cereals, peas, dried beans, meat, milk	Toxicity: hypermagnesemia Deficiency: hypomagnesemia
Iron	Liver, meat, egg yolks, beans, clams, peaches, whole or enriched grains, legumes	Toxicity: hemochromatosis Deficiency: anemia
Copper	Liver, shellfish, nuts, dried legumes, poultry, whole-grain cereals	Toxicity: Wilson's disease Deficiency: anemia

From the NURSE'S REFERENCE LIBRARY volume Diagnostics, published by Intermed Communications, Inc., Springhouse, Pa. 1981.

DIRECTORY OF HELPFUL ORGANIZATIONS

Al-Anon Family Group Headquarters
1 Park Ave.
New York, N.Y. 10016

Alateen World Service Headquarters
1 Park Ave.
New York, N.Y. 10016

Alcoholics Anonymous (AA)
General Service Board of Alcoholics
Anonymous
468 Park Ave., S.
New York, N.Y. 10016

American Association of Diabetes Educators
(AADE)
Box 56
North Woodbury Rd.
Pitman, N.J. 08071

American Association of Sex Educators,
Counselors and Therapists (AASECT)
5010 Wisconsin Ave., N.W.
Washington, D.C. 20016

American Cancer Society (ACS)
777 3rd Ave.
New York, N.Y. 10017

Association for Children with Retarded Mental
Development (A/CRMD)
902 Broadway
New York, N.Y. 10010

American Diabetes Association (ADA)
600 5th Ave.
New York, N.Y. 10020

American Foundation for the Blind (AFB)
15 W. 16th St.
New York, N.Y. 10011

American Red Cross (ARC)
17th and D Sts., N.W.
Washington, D.C. 20006

American Rheumatism Association (ARA)
% Arthritis Foundation
3400 Peachtree Rd., N.E.
Atlanta, Ga. 30326

American Speech-Language-Hearing
Association
10801 Rockville Pike
Rockville, Md. 20852

Anorexia Nervosa and Associated Disorders
(ANAD)
550 Frontage Rd., Suite 2020
Northfield, Ill. 60093

Arthritis Foundation (AF)
3400 Peachtree Rd., N.E.
Atlanta, Ga. 30326

Center for Disease Control
1600 Clifton Rd., N.E.
Atlanta, Ga. 30333

Committee to Combat Huntington's Disease
(CCHD)
250 W. 57th St., Suite 2016
New York, N.Y. 10019

Cystic Fibrosis Foundation
6000 Executive Blvd., Suite 309
Rockville, Md. 20852

Epilepsy Foundation of America (EFA)
1828 L St., N.W., Suite 406
Washington, D.C. 20036

Herpetics Engaged in Living Productively
(HELP)
260 Sheridan Ave.
Palo Alto, Calif. 94306

International Association of Laryngectomees
(IAL)
% American Cancer Society
777 3rd Ave.
New York, N.Y. 10017

Juvenile Diabetes Foundation (JDF)
23 E. 26th St.
New York, N.Y. 10010

Muscular Dystrophy Association, Inc.
810 7th Ave.
New York, N.Y. 10019

Myasthenia Gravis Foundation
15 E. 26th St.
New York, N.Y. 10010

National Foundation—March of Dimes
1275 Mamaroneck Ave.
White Plains, N.Y. 10605

National Hemophilia Foundation (NHF)
25 W. 39th St.
New York, N.Y. 10018

National Huntington's Disease Association
(NHDA)
1441 Broadway, Suite 501
New York, N.Y. 10018

National Lupus Erythematosus Foundation
(NLEF)
5430 Van Nuys Blvd., Suite 206
Van Nuys, Calif. 91401

National Multiple Sclerosis Society (NMSS)
205 E. 42nd St.
New York, N.Y. 10017

National Neurofibromatosis Foundation
340 E. 80th St.
New York, N.Y. 10021

National Parkinson Foundation (NPF)
1501 N.W. 9th Ave.
Miami, Fla. 33136

National Retinitis Pigmentosa Foundation
(NRPF)
Rolling Park Bldg.
8331 Mindale Circle
Baltimore, Md. 21207

National Psoriasis Foundation
6415 Southwest Canyon Court, Suite 200
Portland, Oreg. 97221

National Reye's Syndrome Foundation (NRSF)
509 Rosemont
Bryan, Ohio 43506

National Society for Autistic Children (NSAC)
1234 Massachusetts Ave., N.W., Suite 1017
Washington, D.C. 20005

National Sudden Infant Death Syndrome
Foundation (NSIDSF)
310 S. Michigan Ave., Suite 1904
Chicago, Ill. 60604

National Tay-Sachs and Allied Diseases
Association (NTSAD)
122 E. 42nd St.
New York, N.Y. 10017

President's Committee on Mental Retardation
Regional Office Bldg. #3
7th & D Sts., S.W.
Washington, D.C. 20201

Reach to Recovery Foundation
% American Cancer Society (ACS)
777 3rd Ave.
New York, N.Y. 10017

Smokenders
37 N. 3rd St.
Easton, Pa. 18042

Spina Bifida Association of America (SBAA)
343 S. Dearborn Ave., Suite 319
Chicago, Ill. 60604

United Cerebral Palsy Associations (UCPA)
66 E. 34th St.
New York, N.Y. 10016

United Ostomy Association
1111 Wilshire Blvd.
Los Angeles, Calif. 90017

United Parkinson Foundation (UPF)
220 S. State St.
Chicago, Ill. 60604

U.S. Committee for the World Health
Organization (USC-WHO)
777 United Nations Plaza, 9A
New York, N.Y. 10017

Women Organized Against Rape
P.O. Box 64
Harrisburg, Pa. 17108

From the NURSE'S REFERENCE LIBRARY volume *Diagnostics*, published by Intermed Communications, Inc., Springhouse, Pa. 1981.

TABLE OF EQUIVALENTS

PENICILLIN UNITS
1 unit = 0.6 mcg penicillin G
1 mg penicillin = 1,667 units

WEIGHTS

APOTHECARY	METRIC	APOTHECARY	METRIC
1 ounce =	31.1 g	1/150 grain =	0.4 mg
15.43 grains =	1 g	1/200 grain =	0.3 mg
1 grain =	60 mg	1/250 grain =	0.25 mg
1/60 grain =	1.0 mg	1/300 grain =	0.2 mg
1/80 grain =	0.8 mg	1/400 grain =	0.15 mg
1/100 grain =	0.6 mg	1/500 grain =	0.12 mg
1/120 grain =	0.5 mg	1/600 grain =	0.1 mg

LIQUID MEASURE

HOUSEHOLD		APOTHECARY		APPROXIMATE METRIC
1 teaspoonful	=	1 fluid dram	=	5 ml
1 tablespoonful	=	4 fluid drams	=	15 ml
2 tablespoonfuls	=	1 fluid ounce	=	30 ml
1 measuring cupful	=	8 fluid ounces	=	240 ml
1 pint	=	16 fluid ounces	=	500 ml
1 quart	=	32 fluid ounces	=	1,000 ml

TEMPERATURE
9 C.° = 5 F.° − 160
Centigrade   Fahrenheit
(C.° x 9/5) + 32 = F.°

Fahrenheit   Centigrade
(F.° − 32) x 5/9 = C.°

METRIC WEIGHT EQUIVALENTS
1 kg = 1,000 g
1 g = 1,000 mg
1 mg = 0.001 g
1 mcg or μg = 0.001 mg

CONVERSIONS
1 oz = 30 g
1 lb = 453.6 g
2.2 lb = 1 kg

METRIC VOLUME EQUIVALENTS
1 liter = 1,000 ml
1 deciliter = 100 ml

From the *Nursing82 Drug Handbook*, published by Intermed Communications, Inc., Springhouse, Pa. 1982.

NOTES

NOTES

NOTES

NOTES

NOTES

NOTES

NOTES

NOTES

Nursing72
Nursing73
Nursing74
Nursing75
Nursing76
Nursing77
Nursing78
Nursing79
Nursing80
Nursing81
Nursing82
Nursing83
Nursing84
Nursing85

©1982 Intermed Communications, Inc.